Neural Combat

Neural Combat

STRATEGIES & TACTICS FOR YOUR WAR WITH PARKINSON'S

Terry Currey

FOREWORD

by John Bertoni, M.D., Ph.D.

© 2016 Terry Currey
in association with
CreateSpace Independent Publishing Platform®
Registered through *Booksinprint.com*®
ISBN-10: 1533157901
ISBN-13: 9781533157904

To Kim:

my *Care Giver*, my *Life Coach*, my *Manager*, my *Cheerleader*, my *Fishing Buddy*, my *Biggest Fan*, my *Kindest Critic*, my *Best Friend*, my *Partner*, my *Advocate*, my *Hero, my Angel* – and long before all of that – first and foremost – my *Love*, my *Wife*.

I only have to live with Parkinson's. You have to live with me – well, you don't have to, but fortunately for me – you do.

Table of Contents

Forward

Terry Currey is a fighter. He trained to fight for his country in the Armed Forces. He is now fighting Parkinson's disease.

Terry Currey is not alone.

There are over 320 million people living in the United States in 2016 (US Census Bureau). Since Parkinson's disease has a lifetime risk of 3% - 4%, there are more than 11 million other Terry Curreys that have or will have Parkinson's disease, too.

All his healthcare providers try to help Terry. His family and friends offer support and all of us who may be ready to help and cheer him on are witnesses to his struggle.

Parkinson's disease is formidable foe. It attacks the brain's ability to send messages using the neurotransmitter dopamine.

Dopamine moves us and motivates us. Without enough dopamine people like Terry begin to shake and slow down and movements are weaker. Yet Terry is powerful still — in the way he moves and motivates us!

As a doctor I have the privilege of witnessing his noble struggle. I am only a coach. It is Terry and the millions like him that inspire us to learn more about treating patients and not just treating diseases. The goal is the highest quality of life for the longest possible time!

In these pages, the careful reader will learn not just about Parkinson's disease, but how to cope with adversity. It is an important lesson for all of us.

John M. Bertoni, M.D., Ph.D.

Dr. Bertoni is a nationally recognized authority on Parkinson's disease. He is a Professor of Neurological Sciences at the University of Nebraska Medical Center and Director of UNMC's Parkinson's Disease Clinic. Dr. Bertoni received his M.D. and Ph.D. in Neurological Sciences from the University of Michigan in Ann Arbor where he also completed his residency in Neurology and his fellowship in Neurochemistry. Before joining UNMC in December 2008, Dr. Bertoni was Chairman of the Department of Neurology at Creighton University Medical Center. He has held academic appointments in Michigan, Texas, Pennsylvania, and Delaware. Dr. Bertoni is currently treating Parkinson's patients and participating in several Parkinson's disease related studies.

CHAPTER 1

After That House Fell on Her Sister...

Inside the Mind of an Afflicted Warrior's Brain

For my 10th birthday, my Grandmother gave me a copy of Lessenberry, Crawford, & Erickson's *20th Century Typewriting, 7th Edition.* I was (yawn) thrilled. What 10-year-old boy *doesn't* want to spend his Saturday mornings sitting at a vintage 1925 model *L. C. Smith* learning the home row keys, A S D F – J K L ;? She stood over me, ruthlessly snapping my fingers with a switch whenever I looked down at my hands. "Next year, you'll get a copy of *Gregg's Shorthand Method,* and you'll learn to take proper dictation." ("*I'll have those ruby slippers, my pretty – and your little dog, too!*") I couldn't wait.

Six months later, Mom told me of Grandma's passing. My first thought was *not* "Oh, no! Now, who will teach me shorthand?" I did inherit the *L. C. Smith,* though. When typewritten English compositions came along, I was able to type them, but not with any speed. Couldn't get over looking at the keys, but for high school and college, I got by. When PC keyboards replaced stenographers, I adapted more easily than a lot of guys my age.

Early in 2007, the third finger on my right hand kept sticking on the LLLLLLLLLLLL key. I tried and tried, but I couldn't make it stop. I'd had spinal surgery five years earlier – discectomy and fusion of my sixth and seventh cervical vertebrae – and the neurosurgeon had predicted, "Within ten years, you'll need the same procedure on C-5/C-6." I figured that the clock had run out, and it was time to get my throat slit, again, so I went to see my GP Doc. "I'm referring you to a Neurologist," he said, casually.

"You mean a Neurosurgeon, right?" I corrected.

"A *Neurologist.* Your facial expression and gait are consistent with Parkinson's disease. I need my diagnosis confirmed. You were in Viet Nam. Ever exposed to *Agent Orange?*"

"Now…" as Paul Harvey was known to say, "…for the rest of the story…"

When he told me that I have Parkinson's disease, the Neurologist didn't simply declare, "You have Parkinson's disease." He took a gentler, indirect approach, saying "You are exhibiting symptoms of *Parkinsonian Syndrome.*" Gradually over the next year, the tremors spread from the ring finger to all of the fingers of my right hand; then, to the hand itself; and finally, my entire lower right arm shook uncontrollably.

I would sit on my hand, trying to hide the tremors from others. I stopped eating in public, because I couldn't control the drooling. One of my co-workers thought it was cute to shout over the cubicle wall, "Hey, Terry. What's shakin'?" Reluctantly, I resigned myself to spending the rest of my life living with Dr. James Parkinson's *Shaking Palsy.*

Because my greatest fear is of the unknown, I asked every physician, surgeon, nurse, neurologist, psychologist, therapist, and medical case manager that I met what I could expect as the disease progressed. No one answered definitively. "Everyone's different," they dodged. It dawned on me that although, collectively, they have observed thousands of sufferers, their perspective is from the "outside, looking in." They know how Parkinson's "looks," but with no actual first-hand experience, they don't really know how it "feels." With the experts hedging on what they either did or didn't know, I turned to the only truly reliable source of knowledge – the Internet. I learned more than I ever wanted to know about *hypokinetic rigid syndrome, paralysis agitans,* and the death of *dopaminergic neurons* in the *substantia nigra.* None of this newfound knowledge quieted my fears. With no small amount of trepidation, I exhumed the history of *Operation Ranch Hand,* resurrecting the chemistry of *Tetrachlorodibenzodioxin* contaminated with a 50% solution of *2,4-Dichlorophenoxyacetic Acid.* As my regurgitating anger reopened old wounds from a wrong war fought the wrong way, I raged at the warrior's lesson learned too late: *"When going into Harm's way, check your six. Harm may be behind you."*

Now, my over-active imagination dreams of a nightmare end-stage scenario. It's not pretty. Everything will take more time and more effort. I will become more easily frustrated as my abilities degenerate. Due to the disease, the medication, or both, my usually friendly personality will become paranoid and belligerent. My once beautiful mind will become demented and useless. My speech will become unintelligible. Walking will be more like stumbling. To by-pass my difficulty in swallowing, I will be fed through a tube. Restrained at the wrists and ankles, my bed-ridden, palsied body will shake uncontrollably while I lie in my own filth until some overworked, underpaid institutional employee gets around to changing my diaper and wiping my wrinkled, rash-riddled ass. Ironically, the same ill-advised, inadequately tested military tactic that brought Parkinson's disease to my door has also left me with *Ischemic Heart* disease. If I'm lucky, my heart will implode and deliver me from the agony and humiliation of an ignominious death.

As I said, that's my unbridled imagination – my nightmare – my emotional **DARK SIDE** which "*...cries 'Havoc!' and lets slip the dogs of war.*" Fear trips that trigger far too easily. Finally, reason prevailed. I realized that both my problem and its solution are in my head. My problem is in my brain. Its solution is in my mind, starting with attitude. Either I spend the rest of my life whining that I got beaned by a 95-MPH fastball; or I pick myself up, dust myself off, step to the plate, and swing to "go yard" – worthy of the unwavering support and encouragement from my loving wife and the caring compassion of my family and friends. I can squander precious time and energy crying over circumstances beyond my control; or I can laugh as I live and thank **GOD** I'm alive. "*Make the call,* **BLUE**."

Without cluttering this narrative with scientific terms, I will share what I have learned about diminishing capabilities caused by progressive brain dysfunction due to dopamine deprivation and the strengths & weaknesses of *Carbidopa Levodopa* (*L-DOPA* – synthetic dopamine) medicinal therapy. Quoting Parkinson from the Preface of his *Essay*[1] –

> "*The...caution with which hypothetical statements are admitted, is in no instance more obvious than in those sciences which more particularly belong to the healing art. It therefore is necessary, that some conciliatory*

---

1. Excerpted from *An Essay on the Shaking Palsy* by James Parkinson, *FGS* – Preface
London: original printed by Whittingham and Rowland, Goswell Street, 1817.
On-line eBook edition produced by the *Project Gutenberg Literary Archive* at
http://www.gutenberg.org/files/23777/23777-h/23777-h.htm, 2007, Irma Spehar, Editor.

explanation should be offered for the present publication: in which, it is acknowledged, that mere conjecture takes the place of experiment; and, that analogy is the substitute for anatomical examination, the only sure foundation for pathological knowledge.

"When, however, the nature of the subject, and the circumstances under which it has been here taken up, are considered, it is hoped that the offering of the following pages to the attention of the medical public, will not be severely censured. The disease, respecting which the present inquiry is made, is of a nature highly afflictive. Notwithstanding which…the unhappy sufferer has considered it as an evil, from the domination of which he had no prospect of escape."

MY INTERPRETATION: *"We should discuss the 'Shaking Palsy.' For now, all I have is 'talk.' My conclusions make sense to me, but I have no empirical data to support them – only personal observations. The medical community should not let the lack of experimentation or anatomical examination dissuade them from giving this essay their most earnest consideration. Those afflicted with this evil disease are suffering without hope."*
– "JP"

In writing this book, I am following Dr. Parkinson's lead. The opinions, hypotheses, and conclusions presented herein are largely based on the personal observations of an unschooled lay person – me – who also happens to suffer from the disease. In that regard, I seek no scientific acclamation. My sole motivation in writing this book is to help other sufferers and their care givers adapt as they battle Parkinson's and its symptoms. Unlike your Docs, I know how PD *"feels."* I have agonized over drooling lips, slurring speech, fumbling fingers, and stumbling footsteps. Graceful recovery from such ungraceful moments can only be found in the persistent determination (another PD) to compel one's own mind to subdue one's own brain rather than fall victim to it.

CHAPTER 2

PD and Me

This book chronicles my experience with Parkinson's. The commentary is often couched in the second person, but I intend neither to prescribe nor suggest steps for fellow sufferers or their care givers to take. I only seek to share what I have learned in the hope of helping others by speaking directly to you. I may, from time to time, refer to fellow sufferers with the use of masculine pronouns. I am sharing my experience – I am a man. Likewise, I may refer to care givers with the use of feminine pronouns. That is because my care giver is my wife, a woman, and that is how I relate to her. I am not going to waste time and brain cycles with a bunch of politically correct pronoun neutering. The gender-narcs will just have to get over it.

I know the fear of not knowing – of asking, begging, for answers from the "experts" who would consistently deflect and defer. For those of you who want to know the harsh truth rather than have sunshine blown up your kilt, I have included what open sourced facts I could verify, and I have shared, in detail, my own experiences with the disease, including coping tactics that I have found to work. If, instead, you truly want sunshine, you can find that, along with the all the sand required to bury your head, at the beach.

To begin – a brief history of Terry:

Baby-boomer; native of Omaha, Nebraska; married, three children, five grandchildren.
U.S. Air Force veteran – Air Traffic Controller (four-year enlistment); Viet Nam service.
BGS, University of Nebraska at Omaha (Business major, Civil Engineering minor).
MBA, University of Nebraska – Lincoln (emphases – Economics & Finance).

Career highlights: Airport Operations, City Management, Corporate Financial Analysis, Technology Sales (including *pattern-recognition neural network* bank card software), Technology Project Management, Amateur League and Intercollegiate Baseball Umpire; Docent at the

Strategic Air Command and Aerospace Museum in Ashland, Nebraska; retired.

Credentials: American Association of Airport Executives, International City/County Management Association, Project Management Institute, Mensan, awarded four U.S. Patents in *Voice Recognition* technology.

Interests: **reading** (fiction – techno-thrillers, e.g. Tom Clancy; non-fiction – theoretical physics, e.g. Stephen Hawking), **writing** (personal opinion essay blog: *Lines Out of the Blue*), **fishing** (we own a bass boat and an RV camper), **travel** (set foot on every continent except Antarctica, which is on my bucket list along with exploring my ancestral roots by touring Scotland's distilleries), **collecting single-malt whiskies**, and **baseball** (umpired for 40+ years – personalized license plate reads "*Blue*").

Medical history: typical childhood diseases – measles, mumps, chicken pox, whooping cough, chronic tonsillitis (tonsils removed at age 3, tags removed at age 10); most serious childhood injury – lacerated right eyelid due to a dog bite. As an adult, other than Parkinson's disease, I suffer from ischemic heart disease. Six stents have been inserted into my coronary arteries. Only other major surgery was the C6/C7 discectomy and fusion. I receive annual flu vaccinations but often have a winter bout with bronchitis due to bronchi weakened by whooping cough and unprotected by tonsils. Only known allergy is to bee venom, which when I was stung at age 5, resulted in anaphylactic shock. I've suffered three concussions, each resulting in a loss of consciousness.

Parkinson's disease: first diagnosed in March, 2007. Symptoms include moderate – severe palsy tremors of my lower right (dominant) arm; a frowning/scowling countenance (Parkinson's mask); gaping mouth; wagging tongue; drooling; difficulty swallowing; unstable balance; difficulty arising from sitting or lying; shuffling gait – little or no arm-swing; slurred speech; left foot toes ball into a fist; rigidity in my legs when pivoting; restless leg syndrome (RLS); lost olfactory sense; degraded savory sense; and infrequent, momentary short-term memory loss while speaking.

Daily medication: *Vitamin B-12* (500 mcg), *Ropinirole HCL* (1mg with each meal), *Carbidopa 25/Levodopa 100 mg* x 2 with each meal + 2 additional as needed). For Heart Disease, I also take a statin, a diuretic (*an unsettling combination of LASIX which is also used to treat pulmonary edema in thoroughbred race horses and POTASSIUM CHLORIDE which is injected in lethal doses for capital executions – talk about "Better Living Through Chemistry"*), an anticoagulant, blood pressure medication, and a multi-vitamin. In all, 19 pills every day. Doses are timed for activities and to avoid adverse drug interaction.

Support network: wife, Kim; daughters, Laura and Melissa and their families; son, Cody; numerous friends and colleagues; special thanks to Frank Bracken, Douglas County Veteran Service Officer, American Legion (Nebraska)

Medical team: U.S. Department of Veterans' Affairs Nebraska/ Western Iowa Healthcare System – VA Hospital staff in Omaha, Nebraska:

Primary attending physician – H. Larry Mitchell, M.D. of *Bryan* and *Saint Elizabeth Regional Medical Centers* in Lincoln, Nebraska

Primary resident physician – *varies on a three-year rotation*

Attending neurologist – John Bertoni, M.D., Ph.D. of *Nebraska Medicine* (*University of Nebraska Medical Center*) in Omaha, Nebraska.

Resident neurologist – *varies on a three-year rotation.*

Attending cardiologist – Amy J. Arouni, M.D. of *CHI Health* (*Creighton University Medical Center*) in Omaha, Nebraska.

Resident cardiologist – *varies on a three-year rotation.*

Personal physician – Michael Giitter, M.D. of *Methodist Health System* in Omaha, Nebraska.

Prognosis: *"PD progression over time is measured using the <u>Unified Parkinson's Disease Rating Scale</u> (UPDRS). Medication improved the prognosis of motor symptoms, but is offset by the long-term undesired effects of L-DOPA, which may progress to a state of high dependency on care givers over 15 years. An individual's age is the best predictor of PD effects. Motor decline rate is greater in those with less impairment at initial diagnosis, while cognitive impairment is seen more in patients over age 70 at symptom onset.*

"Disability is not directly related to disease progression. Initially, motor functions are disabled. Since medicinal therapies ease motor symptoms, more non-motor functions are disabled, early on. As PD advances, motor impairments result more from resistance to medication (i.e. speech/swallowing struggles and gait/balance problems), which manifest in 50% of cases after 5 years of L-DOPA usage. After ten years, disability increases due

to autonomic disruptions – insomnia, mood swings, and cognitive decline.

"PD mortality ratios are twice those of normal people. Risk factors include cognitive decline, dementia, old age at onset, and difficulty swallowing. A disease pattern typified by tremor rather than rigidity predicts improved survival. Fatal aspiration pneumonia is twice as common in PD sufferers."

— THE NATURAL HISTORY OF PARKINSON'S DISEASE – *Poewe, U.S. National Library of Medicine, December, 2006*

I am a congenital smart-ass – class clown – always have been. Don't intend to change at this late date. I feel a certain catharsis in self-deprecating humor about my condition. You will find my paltry attempts at humor sprinkled throughout my writing. I mean no offense to my fellow sufferers, nor will I tolerate derision from the able-bodied at the expense of the afflicted. I simply use humor as a defense mechanism – my frightened effort to keep the ominous beast – the unknown – on the other side of the door.

Specifically, I am afflicted with acquired, tremor-dominant Parkinson's disease (PD). Lacking the requisite production of dopamine, my brain's motor functions are stymied. I know how I am supposed to move, but something "blocks" the neural pathways to the intended maneuver. I can almost "feel" that blockade. *L-DOPA* medication temporarily relieves these invisible, non-specific constraints with some "return to normalcy."

Statistically, I am one of a million Americans and seven million people worldwide who suffer from the disease. Most are over 60 years of age. 60% of those are male – predominantly white. About 60,000 Americans are diagnosed each year. Although the disease, itself, is not fatal, about 80,000 – 100,000 deaths annually are attributed to complications derived from PD. *Fatal falls, pulmonary aspiration, deep vein thrombosis,* and *pulmonary embolism* are the most common.

Early stages are effectively treated with medication, but over time, the brain becomes resistant to medicinal therapy. Deep brain stimulation (DBS) is an option for later stages, but that requires invasive surgery to place an electronic device deep inside your brain (hence the name, _deep brain s_timulation). DBS benefits vary, as do their windows of effectiveness. Quite frankly, the thought of an OJT neurosurgery resident at the VA Hospital trolling through my _mesencephalon_ for the purpose of wrapping some kind of _dopaminergic_ shock collar around my _substantia nigra_ scares the _boo-ca-ca_ outta me. For now, I refuse to take the risk, but ask me, again, in ten years.

One caveat: there are some impairments that are gender-specific. I am a man nearing my 70th year. I wear men's clothing. I shave my face, comb my hair, and use the toilet as I have done for my entire life – as a male. When I address tactics that are skewed entirely to the male perspective, I will identify them and apologize to the ladies for being no help in these areas. Any female PD sufferers who want to share their feminine perspective on these topics are welcome to do so. Your contributions will be appreciated.

CHAPTER 3

Logistics

Attitude
Care Givers
Logistical Support Team
Friends & Family

Attitude

You are in a war – not for your life (don't kid yourself – you've already lost that war). No, in this war, you'll battle daily for *TIME*. Without medication, PD sufferers become chair-bound and bed-ridden in as few as eight years after symptom onset. Dementia can set in after ten years. Your goal is to beat the clock. With the right battle tactics, you may be able to double the quality time that you have left to live, love, and pursue happiness. Before you get all dreamy-eyed thinking about loving and pursuing happiness, focus – you're in a war. You will have to fight for every extra day – every extra hour – every extra minute. Also, while there's time, there's hope. The more time you give yourself, the more time you give researchers to find better treatments – maybe even find a cure.

So *lock & load*. This is now your main job – not just for yourself, but for those who love you and whom you love in return. As much as they may want to help you, they can't. Some may lovingly try to "*fix*" you. They can't. Each day's battle will be pitched in *your* head – *your* mind vs. *your* brain. No one else can fight your fight. You, alone, are the sole combatant – on either side. No armor – no weapons, and the field of battle is your body. I'm writing this book to share my coping strategies and tactics in the hope that they will help you develop those of your own unique design to fit your own unique circumstances. The Docs are right – everyone is different, with different symptoms that manifest differently in varying levels of severity. My tactics may not work on your symptoms. You must develop your own tactics for each of your own symptoms. I can only show you what I do. Your mind needs your tactics to fight your brain for control of your body. Ya gotta believe in yourself. If you don't, no one else will.

Care Givers
"…for better or worse – in sickness and in health…"

Because I am familiar with only one style of care giving, I can only relate one style – that of my wife, Kim. Care givers are special people, and if I were granted one wish for my fellow Parkinson's sufferers, it would be that each of their care givers would be like her.

She is eleven years my junior. In addition to being a wife, a mother, and a grandmother; she is businesswoman who has worked outside the home her entire adult life. Of the utmost integrity, diligent in her commitments, and a hard worker, she tolerates no slack effort in herself or those with whom she interacts. A practicing Christian, she is devoted to her family. A wine connoisseur and a gourmet chef, she attended the *Institute for Culinary Arts* in Omaha. She sets a high bar for herself, which she rarely fails to clear.

As for dealing with my Parkinson's, she views it as a partnership. She expects me to participate as a full partner and face my challenges by providing as much care for myself as I can muster. She asks that I help where I can with household chores – laundry, meal clean-up, yard work, etc. She absolutely will not allow me to use Parkinson's as an excuse for not doing what she believes I can do and is quick to chastise me when she thinks I am making excuses. By steadfastly encouraging me to take a positive outlook, she insists that I refuse to let the disease define me as an individual; nor will she allow it to define us as a couple. She stays fully informed on my medication regimen and sees that I follow it. She keeps me actively engaged with family and friends. We travel a couple of times each year and take short fishing & camping excursions most weekends, weather permitting. She plans and organizes all of that. I can still drive, so I transport myself around town or to my part-time job and share the driving on long auto trips. She spends workdays at her office. Before leaving the house, she ensures that what I need for that day's activities is either readily available or within my ability to obtain. Except for her workday, we are together most of the time. She stays aware of where I am and what I am doing. She has an uncanny sixth sense that, upon seeing me struggle with a task, tells her when to intervene and when to let me work through it.

No stranger herself to pain, she is moderately afflicted with rheumatoid arthritis, which has worsened with age. She self-treats it with activity, exercise, diet, and an occasional OTC pain reliever; but it is simply not her style to burden others with complaints. She is both an example for and an inspiration to me. In short – I love her, and I admire her.

If she seems perfect, she isn't. Far from it, she is human. She has her own bad days as a result of either my declining health or hers – or both. Watching the man she loves, admires, and has relied upon for most of our marriage become progressively dysfunctional saddens her, greatly. Reluctantly, she marks that progression each time that I am no longer able to perform some routine task – one more frustrating thing that either she must do or find a way to get done. On occasion, her frustration turns to anger. Far too dignified to express that anger openly, she reserves those moments for when we are alone, and she can control her emotions. She is never abusive with her temper and, to her credit, insists that we confront whatever issue we are facing by talking our way through it, not allowing me to withdraw behind the wall of my own psyche. She shares my fear of the dark, unknown future.

We are both aware that the time is coming when I will be totally dependent on her or (more likely, given that she is the primary breadwinner) on an in-home professional for my day-to-day care, and we have prepared for that eventuality. What neither of us can prepare to face is the day when she must commit me to a permanent care facility and forego our time together. We simply trust in God, take what each day brings, and try not to think that far ahead. Whenever self-pity gets the better of me and I think my life is hard, I need only remind myself that without her, I would have no life at all. Parkinson's notwithstanding – she is my love, my wife, my life.

Logistical Support Team

In addition to your care giver and medical team, you may need urgent or emergency assistance when your care giver is not available. Response for this need requires –

1. a personal, hand-held, mobile communications device with you at all times;
2. a network team of individuals – family members, friends, neighbors – willing to respond, 24/7, to urgent (non-emergency) calls for assistance;
3. 24-hour telephone numbers for team members programmed into "speed dial" on the mobile communications device in order of contact priority (i.e. Speed Dial #1 => highest priority contact, SD #2 => second highest priority contact, etc.);

4. for emergency assistance (injury or threat to life) ***CALL 9-1-1***. You may want to alert nearby first responders to your situation and home location;

5. a procedure that notifies your support team network when you plan to travel by car, alone, more than 50 miles from home;

6. a procedure that ensures that a team member checks on your safety whenever severe weather, criminal activity, or civil unrest threatens your location;

7. a notification procedure that alerts the network of planned absences when network team members will not be available;

8. a list of network team contact information distributed to each member; and

9. medication instructions and healthcare provider contacts for each team member.

This often overlooked aspect of living with PD is essential to the sufferer's well-being. Appropriate, timely response to requests for assistance can mean the difference in keeping a need to resolve an otherwise simple problem from becoming a threat to life or limb. You can manage your reactions to the challenges of PD, but you can't do it alone.

Friends & Family

All analyses begin with an enumerated set of conditions that are assumed as *"given."* They comprise the baseline – the "facts" of the case. Interactive relationships and hypothetical variations can be construed from that base, but the foundation remains solid.

The support you receive from those people who are close to you is also solid – to quote Bob Seeger, "...*like a* ROCK." Although you can take that as *"given,"* you must *never* "...take it for granted." Sounds contradictory, doesn't it? It's not. What they give to you in support and encouragement, they give out of love, respect, and compassion. There is neither obligation on their part nor entitlement on yours. You need them more than they need you. Never forget that. They and their gifts must be cherished and protected.

Protected? From what?

From you and your brain. You must guard them against some sudden outburst of frustration resulting from your inability to execute what used to be the simplest of tasks. You must remember that they don't know how Parkinson's "feels." They only know how it "looks." Some of them may see you only during brief, infrequent visits. The miniscule, imperceptible, day-by-day changes to your appearance, demeanor, and abilities are compounded over the time between those visits. Shield them from the shock.

SMILE. BE NICE.

If you're greeted with "*Hey – how's it goin'? Gosh, you look great!*" They don't need the gory details. Smile – swap lies with 'em. "*Never better. I've always been good looking.*"

CHAPTER 4

Paralysis Agitans

(Latin: *Shaking Palsy*)

Pattern Recognition
Connecting the Dots

I.   *Systemic Functions* ≅ *Supporting Infrastructure*
II. *Sensory Perception* ≅ *Data Entry/Input*
III. *Forms of Expression* ≅ *Output*
IV. *Cognitive Functions* ≅ *Central Processing Logic*

Pattern Recognition

For those who are struggling to grasp what is happening to them, I will try to explain Parkinson's disease as I understand it. Mine is a layman's view of a highly complex and largely unexplained problem, _chemical deficiency_, which adversely impacts a highly complex and largely unexplored environment, the human brain. I am neither a neurologist nor any type of healthcare professional. I am blessed with a high intellectual capacity, but my education of human brain functions is limited to my high-school biology class (50+ years ago) and what I can glean from impromptu forays into _Wikipedia_. My graduate education is oriented toward business, economics, and engineering.

Although I have a lifetime of experience with automated Information Technology (IT), it is from a _business_ perspective of information services – technology corporate finance, technology sales, and technology project management. My formal computer science education consists of three semesters of _FORTRAN_ programing language (circa 1966). At best, I have gained a strong working knowledge of IT systems and processes.

So find a quiet spot, curl up, and get comfy. Put all sharp objects well out of reach. Have something heavily caffeinated close at hand. You're gonna need it. Have another nice something like a fine single-malt _whisky_ ready at the other end, if you're still conscious.

There's just no simple way to explain this stuff. It involves algebra, physics, chemistry, biology, medicine, neurology, information technology, and every now and then, some Latin may be thrown in. Don't you wish you had paid attention to all that crap you blew off in high school? If you get lost, have _Google_ or _Siri_ handy. I could try to "dumb it down," but that would be counterintuitive. As I state later in the book, stretching your cognitive abilities will delay dementia, so saddle up. Here comes the skull stretcher.

Unless you're a nerd, like me, you won't enjoy this chapter. Most likely, it will bore you. It may frighten you – worst case, you'll find it incomprehensible. Read it, anyway. It's like the mushy green vegetables of the book – tastes yukky, but good for you. Marketing and pharmaceutical company execs are excused because, as we all know, "Real men don't do numbers." (I was almost hired as the CEO of a pharmaceutical company, but I blew the interview when I passed the intelligence test.) Ba-dump-bump...

Programmed by the finger of God, the human brain is the most elegant computer ever devised. It is dynamic – ever-changing – more so than any other organ. Like software updates and upgrades that revise and refresh Operating Systems, Firmware, User Interfaces, and Applications; our dynamic brains reflect life's ever-changing conditions. Humans grow, develop skills, acquire knowledge, experience events, learn, discern, distinguish, deliberate, memorize, contemplate, communicate, imagine, socialize, adapt, age, and ultimately – die. Throughout our lives, our brains stimulate our actions, enable their execution, and record the outcomes. As difficult as change may be for some folks, it is essential to our existence. Without change, there is no growth. Without growth, there can be no life. The Marine Corps dictum, "*Improvise! Adapt! Overcome!*" says it best.

The human brain is governed by a cognitive learning process known as *Pattern Recognition*. All data gathered through our conscious sensory perception systems and our subconscious autonomic physiological systems are assimilated, categorized, and organized into data pattern arrays; which are cataloged, indexed, and stored for future use in recognizing new incoming patterns and employing recognized patterns for outgoing task execution. Anthropologists speculate that the survival of the species, Homo sapiens, is due in large part to a keenly conditioned "*fight-or-flight*" response instigated by this precisely structured system of recognized patterns. Having sold and managed projects installing machine-virtual, neural-network, bank card fraud detection systems; I am familiar with three generations of machine-virtual pattern recognition capabilities:

1st Gen – artificial intelligence – basic "*...if, then...*" and "*...either, or...*" Boolean decision-making.
2nd Gen – expert systems – pattern models which require extensive human intervention to train and update.

3rd Gen – neural networks – pattern models which, once trained, are capable of very simple intrinsic updates.

Connecting the Dots

To illustrate, a computerized pattern recognition system has three constituents: a _pattern model_ consisting of _multiple recognized data pattern arrays_ and an _unrecognized incoming data pattern array_.

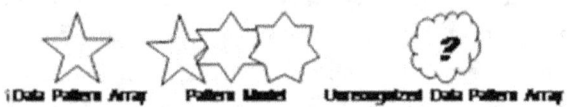

i Data Pattern Array   Pattern Model   Unrecognized Data Pattern Array

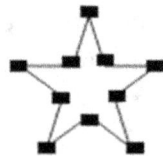

The data pattern array has two components: pattern data points (depicted as dots) and the linear or non-linear mathematical relationships among the data (depicted as lines). Connect the dots with lines to construct the pattern array.

Current state neural networks don't learn in a human sense. More precisely, they emulate human learning by applying an adaptation of Dr. Leon Cooper's[2] complex _Probabilistic Restricted Coulomb Energy_ algorithm. When 3rd Gen neural networks were first introduced, system constraints (primarily i/o throughput capacity) made pattern arrays with greater than eight data points infeasible. This is a direct result of the geometric progression in the number of relationships when a single datum is added to the array.

Each member of a group relates to every other member of that group; therefore in a group (a/k/a _data pattern array_) of **n** members (a/k/a _data points_), each member has potentially (**n** -1) intra-group relationships. If the relationships are bi-directional (i.e. A $\longleftrightarrow$ B), the total number of _potential_ relationships in the group = $\frac{n(n-1)}{2}$. However if, as is the case with neural networks,

---

2. Leon N. Cooper, Ph.D. – _Thomas J. Watson, Sr. Professor of Science_ and _Director of the Institute for Brain and Neural Systems_ at Brown University who, along with John Bardeen and John Schrieffer was awarded the 1972 Nobel Prize in Physics for developing the _BCS Theory of Superconductivity_.

the group's relationships are uni-directional (i.e. A ⇌ B), the total number of *potential* relationships in the group = $n (n -1)$.

Not all relationships within a data pattern array are fulfilled, which creates a natural distinction between two pattern arrays with the same data points. For example, bank card transactions from two different cardholders of the same bank may have the same data points in their card usage pattern arrays such as *transaction amount, merchant, geographic location, merchandise purchased*, and *transaction timestamp*; but because the cardholders are two differently behaving individuals, the mathematical relationships within their respective data pattern arrays will populate differently. B-T-W, this is only one of a multitude of ways in which your electronic persona is tracked and trended. We are way beyond *1984*, and **BIG BROTHER** is definitely watching.

Eight data points in a neural network data pattern array yields 56 potential relationships. Add one data point to the array, and the number of potential relationships jumps to 72. Add another and the relationship count is 90. In an IT environment, adding relationships adds i/o throughput time. Eventually, adding one data point overloads the throughput capacity and brings the whole process to its knees. Hypothetically, the process could benefit with the addition of a streamlining algorithm such as *Karmarkar*,[3] but even with such an enhancement which would increase the number of manageable data point variables in a machine environment from seven or eight to more than seven or eight thousand, that still comes nowhere near the pattern recognition capacity of the human brain.

If we were to infer a human brain pattern recognition neural net structure from the IT example (not sure that such an inference is valid, except, maybe, as an illustration), the "dots" would be neurons, and the "lines" would be synapses. Now, the analogy weakens: each neuron connects to over 60,000 other neurons, and our brains have over *100 MILLION* neurons. If we apply the relationship math from our IT example, we calculate the human brain's pattern array capacity at over *TEN QUADRILLION* (that's 10 followed by 15

---

3. Karmarkar's algorithm, introduced by Narendra Karmarkar in 1984, was the first reasonably efficient algorithm to solve linear programming problems in polynomial time.

zeros) potential relationships! If the calculation is off by a factor of 100,000, that's still lightyears beyond the largest, fastest machine capability.

The point of all of this mega-math is to emphasize the mission-critical role of the brain chemical, *dopamine*. Picture all of these data-point neurons networked with one another by their linear/non-linear-relationship synapses and organized into data pattern arrays cataloged in a vast library within the brain to enable everything from simple nutrient digestion to complex conceptualization. Dopamine acts as librarian/guide, mapping neural pathways to access patterns required to execute tasks. Without dopamine, our motor and cognitive brain functions are stymied when attempting to access the pattern library in search of the pattern arrays needed for task execution.

The production of dopamine doesn't stop suddenly, overnight. It dwindles at an insidiously slow rate. So slowly that, in the beginning, most sufferers don't notice the very slight, subtle changes in their body's motor, sensory, or cognitive functions. This trickling deterioration in brain function is what gives the disease its apparent progressive (rather than degenerative) character. Imagine a mass of millions of dopaminergic neuron cells producing dopamine in sufficient quantities for the brain to function normally. Then, slowly – ever so slowly, the mass of cells begins to deplete – as the cells die, one or two at-a-time – with the dead cells being eliminated from the body, and no new cells being generated to replace them. Miniscule, barely noticeable breakdowns in motor, sensory, and cognitive control begin to occur – sporadically, at first; then gradually, with greater frequency and dysfunction. Finally, the cellular loss reaches critical mass, the brain goes rogue, and full-blown Parkinson's disease manifests with its myriad symptoms.

During the early-to-middle stages, medicinal therapy (L-DOPA) compensates for the declining chemical production. As more and more dopamine-producing cells die, sufferers are forced to concentrate harder and harder to execute the simplest movements – blinking, swallowing, walking, etc. Medication helps, but eventually, the brain's dopaminergic cellular loss is too overwhelming, and meds are powerless to offset the deficit.

I view the brain as a "shared resource." I don't know if the field of Neurology has considered (or recognizes) the concept of shared resources. Fictional sentient androids (e.g. *The Terminator*, Data in *ST:NG*, or Ash and Bishop in the *Alien* series) are anthropomorphized machines with humanoid features. Films such as *Defending Your Life* and *LUCY* or the TV series, *Limitless*, hypothesize humans consciously increasing control of their brain functions. Clearly, such plots do not consider shared resource limitations.

To me, the notion of conscious human control of 100% of the brain would be analogous to one DSL user sucking up all of the bandwidth by streaming kitten videos, thereby impeding access to the network by other users. The brain's primary "users" are the body's *conscious motor, subconscious motor, autonomic physiological, subconscious psychological,* and *conscious cognitive* functions. Much like a computer, each requires adequate work space. IT platform sizing is a function of both *data storage* capacity and *CPU i/o throughput* capacity. Work spaces are based on field length, record size, periodic volume, periodic frequency distribution, and storage interval; *plus* necessary space for memory, back-up, growth, system overhead, and related ancillary applications.

I believe that the brain's pattern management capacity is similarly apportioned. I offer an observation that seems, on the surface, to support my contention. A disproportionate number of my Mensa group ($\approx$25%) suffer from some acquired or congenital, non-traumatic physical disability or neurological disorder: ADHD, Tourette's, Parkinson's, Asperger's, MS, impaired sensory perception, partial paralysis, etc. Theoretical physicist, Stephen Hawking – an Amyotrophic Lateral Sclerosis (ALS) sufferer – is another and, probably, the most prominent example. It is as if the brain is a finite capacity resource, and if an extravagant amount of that capacity is usurped by higher intellectual demands – well, "*somethin's gotta give.*"

Most people (myself included) are unfamiliar with neurological terminology. Conversely, "smart" phones have exposed the masses to IT terminology. To further illustrate the similarities between machine information processing and human brain functions, I have mapped the various human brain functions to their IT counterparts.

From my lay person's perspective, the functional categories of recognized patterns and their equivalent IT system counterparts include –

1. ***Internally imposed patterns*** ≅ ***binary machine language.*** "Factory installed" autonomic motor function patterns over which the conscious, unconscious, or subconscious mind has no control – i.e. digestion, circulation, respiration, etc.
2. ***Internally developed patterns*** ≅ ***firmware.*** Appropriate implementation of these patterns are recognized as the individual matures. They include subconscious processes along with physiological and psychological states.
3. ***Internally developed patterns*** ≅ ***operating system.*** These patterns relate to basic muscle movement and sensory functions.
4. ***Acquired patterns*** ≅ ***message transport layer.*** Recognized patterns that carry instructions from the pattern library to the intended motor function.
5. ***Acquired patterns*** ≅ ***operating system.*** Recognized patterns that enable interpretation of perceived sensations.
6. ***Acquired patterns*** ≅ ***user interface.*** Recognized patterns that enable communication between intellectual processes and purposeful motor functions.
7. ***Acquired patterns*** ≅ ***application layer.*** Recognized patterns that enable interaction among perceptive, cognitive, and expressive functions.

My descriptions of pattern recognition, neural networks, and my characterization of dopamine as a sort of combined "gate keeper – librarian – traffic cop – neural pathfinder" are unconventional, overly simplified, and maybe even naïve. They are inferred conjecture. I offer them to PD sufferers and their care givers who may be unfamiliar with medical and IT terminology or academic research. I tried to keep the footnotes to a minimum.

My depictions may be unorthodox, but that doesn't mean they're wrong. Do I understand them? Yes. Can I prove them? No. Like Parkinson with his *Essay*, I'm too old, too disabled, and too tired to undertake such an exhaustive task. Let someone younger, more capable, with brighter eyes and a bushier tail chase that paper. I ask the scientific and academic communities is to step outside their respective boxes and consider a lay person's view, remembering that all research begins with the same three words: *"I don't know."* Just give my name an "honorable mention" when accepting your Nobel Prize.

To further illustrate my *"machine-virtual neural network comparison with human brain neural network"* analogy, I have grouped human physiological and cognitive functions into their (roughly) corresponding IT functional categories.

I. Systemic Functions ≅ Supporting Infrastructure

    A. Autonomic Processes (internally imposed patterns – binary machine language)

1.	Digestion	7.	Unconscious activity (e.g. dreaming)
2.	Energy conversion		
3.	Respiration	8.	Growth
4.	Circulation	9.	Regeneration
5.	Perspiration	10.	Aging
6.	Elimination	11.	Others

    B. Subconscious Processes (internally developed patterns – firmware)

1.	Blinking	5.	Pattern filtering
2.	Swallowing	6.	Pattern library cataloging
3.	Physical balance	7.	Others
4.	Elimination control		

    C. Physiological States (internally developed patterns – firmware)

1.	Fatigue	7.	Fever
2.	Vigor	8.	Chill
3.	Pain	9.	Nausea
4.	Hunger	10.	Physical disabilities
5.	Thirst	11.	Neurological disorders
6.	Satiation	12.	Others

D. Psychological States (internally developed patterns – firmware)
1. Emotions
2. Phobias
3. Psychoses
4. Preferences
5. Aversions
6. Personality
7. Temperament
8. Conditioned responses
9. Behavior
10. Others

II. Sensory Perception ≅ Data Entry/Input
(internally developed patterns – operating system)

A. Stereoscopic vision
B. 360° hearing
C. Tactile sense
D. Savory sense
E. Olfactory sense

III. Forms of Expression ≅ Output

A. Linguistic formulation
B. Musical articulation
C. Artistic endeavor
D. Social interaction
E. Cognitive conceptualization
F. Others

IV. Cognitive Functions ≅ Central Processing Logic

A. Consciously Coordinated Motor Processes (acquired patterns – operating system)
1. Bipedal ambulation
2. Manual dexterity
3. Linguistic communication
4. Purposeful expression
5. Energy management – reserve, use, restore
6. Physical exertion
7. Physical attitude (lying, standing, sitting, etc.)
8. Others

B. Neural Network (acquired patterns – message transport layer)
1. Neurons ≅ random access memory-bit location addresses
2. Synapses ≅ circuitry – virtual and physical

3. Memory patterns ≅ virtual shapes defined by points (neurons) connected by circuits (synapses)
4. Nervous system ≅ Local Area Network

C. Intellectual Processes (acquired patterns – application layer)
1. Short-term memory ≅ Random Access Memory
2. Long-term memory ≅ Direct Access Storage Disc
3. Sentient interaction ≅ (no comprehensive machine equivalent – yet)
   a. pattern perception
   b. pattern realization
      1) pattern awareness   3) pattern manipulation
      2) pattern assimilation   4) pattern organization
   c. pattern recognition
   d. pattern conceptualization
   e. pattern composition
   f. pattern expression

This book describes motor dysfunctions common among Parkinson's sufferers and the compensatory tactics I use to overcome them. With each, I included my assumptions regarding the recognized patterns' origins and equivalent IT functional machine layers.

OK. You can relax, now. The hard part is over. Pour the scotch.

CHAPTER 5

Upside, Downside, Bright Side, DARK Side

Personality and Temperament (internally developed patterns – firmware)

This a double-whammy. Seems that the dark changes to a PD sufferer's personality and in his temperament are both side-effects of the medication and symptoms of the disease, itself. I hesitate to over-simplify, but this whole issue boils down to a first-grade Sunday School lesson: *The Golden Rule*. Be vigilant – watch your words, your tone, your manner, and your behavior. Go to extremes to be helpful, kind, and considerate. In fact, read and re-read the *Boy Scout Handbook*. Skip knot tying. Focus on the stuff about being *Helpful, Courteous, Kind, Brave, Loyal, Trustworthy*, etc. Look around. Who's with you? Why are they there? Because they feel sorry for you? Not likely. All of the pity people bailed a long time ago. The folks that are left? They care about you, or they care *for* you, or they are foolish enough to *love* you. Don't hurt *them*, or you'll have a much shorter life, ending in a lonely death. Be nice.

Emotional Reactions (internally developed patterns – firmware)

> *"Dear Lord:*
> *Please grant me the serenity to accept the things I cannot change, the courage to change the things I can, and the wisdom to know the difference."*
> — THE SERENITY PRAYER

Prepare yourself to repeatedly encounter the full range of your emotions. You will experience *love, gratitude, elation, humiliation, frustration, anxiety, anger, hurt, grief,* among others and, of course, the **DARK SIDE** – *self-pity* and *fear*. They are unavoidable human nature. You may encounter one emotion several times in one day. You may encounter multiple emotions simultaneously. The main thing to remember is DON'T PANIC. Go ahead – experience your emotions. Emotions are meant to be experienced. They are part of the process we call "life." Just don't let them consume you. Of course, you're depressed. That's part of your fading cranial landscape, but resist the use of another medicinal solution to regain your composure. Contrary to that 1950s slogan hoisted by the advertising geniuses at DuPont, chemistry is not necessarily the pathway to "better living." Your brain may be out of control, but you still hold the reins on your mind. You cannot change your brain dysfunction. You must accept that. You can control your reactions to your symptoms. At times, that will take courage. Gather wisdom about what you *feel* and how you *think*, then learn when to do which.

The Highs – love, gratitude, elation, etc.
Feeling good feels good, but don't overdo it. The higher you get, the farther you fall when the good times end. Limit risk by limiting exposure. Control your emotions by constraining them to moderation. It's OK to let yourself experience strong feelings, but don't let any feelings – good or bad – control you. Keep one foot grounded in reason.

The Lows – humiliation, frustration, anxiety, anger, hurt, grief, etc.
The same can be said for the bad times. Don't allow yourself to get so low that you can't climb out. Limit the amount of time that you allow yourself to feel badly – 10 or 15 minutes. Then, engage in some activity that will result in a positive outcome, and move on. Ensure that these negative emotions are not only controlled but also contained – especially anger. Do not allow them to spill up all over anyone else. Personality and temperament changes are both symptoms of the disease and side effects of the medication. An even temper and a friendly personality may require extra concentration on your part. Be extra vigilant to be on your best behavior. Yes, the symptoms of the disease can be humiliating, frustrating, and hurtful. That's no one's fault. If you take out your anger on those around you, the only thing you will accomplish is to hurt someone else – probably someone close to you. Then, you get to experience *regret, guilt, remorse* and *shame* for having allowed your emotional state of mind to lead you to behave so badly that you hurt another. Your brain wins.

Self-pity (acquired patterns – application layer)
This is the poorest, most non-productive use of precious time and waning energy that I know. It is practically impossible to move forward while looking

back. Yes, you got a raw deal. No, it isn't fair. Get over it. You're wasting time. Look around. People in predicaments much worse than the one you're in are doing much more than you are. Grow up. Decide, now, how you're going to live the rest of your life – as a victim or as a survivor.

Fear (internally developed patterns – firmware)
The best way to deal with fear is to face it. Identify precisely what you fear. Give it a name. Then educate yourself on the various causes and effects of that fear. What will cause it to become reality? What will the impact be to you – to your loved ones – to the planet – to the universe? What is the probability of this fear becoming a reality? If the probability is high, can it be prevented? How? What are the steps to prevention?

Rate your fears from 1 (least fearsome) to 10 (most fearsome). Estimate the potential exposure, impact magnitude, and probability of occurrence. Develop mitigation strategies for the top three. Understanding fear demystifies it. Quantifying a fear raises the curtain that hides it, illuminates the demon, and gives it a structure that you can master. Journal your fears and their respective assessments. Conduct regular reality checks.

Yes, there will be good days and bad days. Good days are wonderful. Bad days suck. In the beginning, your good days will far outnumber your bad days. You'll almost forget that you have Parkinson's. You'll do normal stuff. You'll be your normal self. Life will be good. Then, without warning – **WHAM!** Bad day. Nothing will go right. Your symptoms will overwhelm you. You'll get dejected, discouraged, and depressed. Allow yourself the luxury of self-pity for 10 minutes – no more than 15, but don't reach for some pill to feel better. You've got enough of those in your life. Pharmaceutical company CEOs are buying vacation homes and putting their kids through Ivy League universities with the money they make from your affliction, so get past the emotion and *THINK*. Recall your worst day. Is this one better or worse?

Better? Well then, you've survived worse – you can survive whatever this day brings.

Worse? OK – a new low benchmark – remember it; commit it to writing for future reference. Make note of the fact that you are still alive, and take heart in the words of German philosopher Friedrich Nietzsche – "*That which defeats you but does not destroy you only makes you stronger.*" Take the strength. Put it in the *WIN* column and move on.

Nothing builds self-confidence like success. Find an achievable goal, make a plan, and follow through. It doesn't have to be monumental. You don't have to build a Cathedral, for crying out loud. Keep it simple. Mow the lawn. Weed the garden. Take a walk. Do twenty minutes on the treadmill. Do one simple thing, so that when you've done it, you can say, "There. I did that." Then, take on the next thing – a little more difficult, and the next, and the next, and so on. Make a list. Check 'em off. With concentration and a modicum of effort, you'll have a string of achievements and maybe – just maybe – you will have turned a bad day into a good one.

Want to feel even better? The best way to get your mind off your problems is to help someone less fortunate. No matter how bad you think your situation is, you can always find someone who is worse off. Volunteer at a vets' hospital. Help an elderly neighbor. You'll be surprised at how much better you will feel. Now, you have stuff to do – friends to visit, people to love, articles to write, concerts to attend, books to read, things to learn, fish to catch, problems to solve – whatever – forget Jimmy Parkinson. Lace up your *Nikes*®, and *JUST DO IT*.

Paranoia (internally developed patterns – firmware)
This is one of *Fear's* many variations. People will make simple, non-threatening inquiries about your physical condition or your state of mind, and you will take offense, complaining that they're intruding in your life – trying to manage your activities or trying to control you.

Lighten up. These folks are concerned about and for you. Remember our **Friends & Family** discussion (page 17) Stop thinking that everyone is out to get you or your assets or that they, somehow, think less of you. If you can't do that, your brain wins. SMILE. BE NICE.

Physical Exercise (acquired patterns – application layer)

Physical therapists, personal trainers, and athletic coaches call it "*muscle memory.*" Until I learned of *pattern recognition*, I figured it was just a training gimmick used to positively reinforce a desired conditioned response. Well, it is exactly that and much more.

From conception (alright – *Pro-Lifers & Pro-Choicers* – back off! We're not going to open that can of worms, here); the human brain assimilates, recognizes, and catalogues patterns of activity. Early stages of gestation involve simple patterns of cell division & growth, DNA configuration, nutrient ingestion, circulation, etc. Later stages involve movement and the beginnings of sentient awareness. Upon leaving the womb, the brain's learning process kicks into high gear. All sensory patterns are unrecognized – sights, sounds, smells, tastes, touches, and their myriad combinations. They must be acquired, cataloged, and stored for future recognition. With consistent reinforcement, intentional action is learned – motion, speech, and other cognitive motor skills. Muscles, tendons, ligaments, and bones develop and strengthen the framework of the human body. At the core of this process is the brain chemical, dopamine, a combination librarian-pathfinder that permits access to and guides through the neural pathway maze to the innumerable cataloged "muscle memory" patterns in the pattern library.

Parkinson's, a neurological disorder, is caused by a lack of dopamine due to the death of the brain cells that produce it, resulting in a gradual degradation of muscle function. Physical exercise will slow that degradation by reinforcing muscle memory patterns and delaying entropy. Walking and lower body strength conditioning will lengthen the time that your leg muscles remain functional and lessen the severity of symptoms like cramping and restless leg syndrome (RLS). Upper body conditioning will do the same for your arms and lessen the severity of tremors. Ask your medical team for either a professionally conducted or a self-guided physical exercise program.

Mental Exercise (acquired patterns – application layer)

The more you strengthen your cognitive ability, the longer you will hold off dementia. Stretch your mind. Become a nerd, if you're not one already. Study theoretical physics or macro-economics. Shun calculators – do life's math problems in your head. Learn to use a slide rule (*Google* it) or a sextant (*Siri?*). Write your memoirs. *Blog.* Learn to play Chess. Join trivia groups. Study the malting and distillation of single-malt *whisky*. Delve into the difficult. Stimulate your imagination. *THINK* – push your mind _hard_.

Although excessive time mindlessly sitting in front a television screen can be harmful, some video games help strengthen hand-eye coordination. I prefer flight simulators, fishing games, and *Jeopardy!* On the other hand, I don't enjoy POV gun-shooting games. Been to actual war. Don't need to simulate it, virtually. Thank you, very much.

Reading is best, though – fiction, non-fiction, or both – it doesn't matter. With no picture tube, your mind is forced to imagine the pictures. Books too clumsy to hold in your shaking hands? Try audiobooks. Professional reader-narrators have a repertoire of voices for each character that gives life to the material. It's like listening to old-time radio.

In reading this book, note that its vocabulary extends well beyond the middle school comprehension level prescribed by most marketing executives for mass communications (*marketing execs – form-over-function spin merchants that gave us the Edsel, "New" Coke, and "4 times less Charmin."*) That is my intent. I'm pushing you. In doing so, I simultaneously stimulate your cognitive abilities _and_ mine. Good for both of us. If there's a concept you don't understand, it's not like you have to search the library card catalogue or *Periodical Index.* You're sitting there reading this with *Google* or *Siri in your other hand!* The only way I could get this stuff into your head faster would be with a *Vulcan Mind Meld.* Live long and prosper.

Purposeful thought is the goal – deductive reasoning, forensic rhetoric, problem solving, mental calculation, topical study, Socratic method, brainstorming, cognitive conceptualization. Share what you learn – mentor others. You don't have to cure cancer, invent the *flux capacitor*, or perfect cold fusion energy. Just *think – create – imagine*. Albert Einstein said, "*Imagination is more important than knowledge. Knowledge is the sum total of everything we know, today. Imagination is the preview of life's coming attractions.*"

CHAPTER 6

Taking Command

Medication Regimen
Symptom Response Tactics
Fatal Complications

Medication Regimen

The best thing that you can do to relieve PD symptoms is to stay on your medication. Stick to a regimented schedule. The meds may cause some gastrointestinal discomfort. The Docs will tell you that the timed-release effect of L-DOPA works best if you take it before a meal, but taking it on an empty stomach may cause indigestion. What you can do is eat a few bites to get food in your belly, then take your meds and finish your meal.

As PD progresses, L-DOPA's effective dosage interval will gradually decrease as your brain builds resistance to the medication. Monitor this interval closely. Learn the warning signs indicating when your meds are "wearing off." Neither increasing the dosage amount or frequency, nor reducing the time between doses will help. Such measures will only serve to compound your brain's resistance. As resistance builds, you will have to endure lengthening periods of being between doses. That's why mastering these symptom response tactics is so critical. When planning an activity that will span multiple medication doses, allow for that "downtime."

Symptom Response Tactics

When the medication is working, everything is glorious. You walk normally. You talk normally. You don't drool. Life is good. About twenty minutes after you take the medication, you will feel this wonderful sensation of calming muscle control wash through your entire body. It is so-o-o soothing. However, there will be times when you will be "off your meds" and alone. The following tactics are suggested to get you through those times.

To ensure that we are not re-inventing the wheel, There are physical therapy clinics that specialize in treating Parkinson's sufferers. For example, you can obtain speech and mobility physical therapy from licensed *LSVT[4] Global®* franchised training clinics, which are endorsed by the National Parkinson's Foundation. When seeking this type of therapy, ask the clinic if they provide the *"LSVT Big"* and/or *"LSVT Loud"* therapies.

---

4 Lee Silverman Voice Treatment

For the uninitiated, able-bodied reader, these coping tactics may seem to be common sense. *"Remember to blink. Close your mouth. Remember to swallow. DUH ! These are things I learned as a child."* Well, DUH right-back-atcha. Yes, these are very elementary tasks, learned as a child. Many are executed as sub-conscious or autonomic brain functions enabled by dopamine. When inadequately medicated, Parkinson's sufferers do not have the benefit of dopamine and must concentrate to execute the simplest of tasks. While concentrating on three simultaneous tasks, a fourth one slips through the net, and the result is drooling or stumbling or something else equally embarrassing. So – PD sufferers and care givers, continue reading. Yes, the reminders sound like admonitions from you Mother: *"Pick up your feet." "Close your mouth." "Take your meds." "Eat your vegetables." "Stand up straight." "Don't talk with your mouth full." "Get up – get out of bed." "Do your chores."* "SMILE." "BE NICE." Anyone else who finds this funny, go ahead – laugh. You're kinda makin' my point.

Fatal Complications

Remember the Big 4 – *deep vein thrombosis (DVT)*, *pulmonary embolism (PE)*, *pulmonary aspiration*, and *fatal falls*? I will offer tactics to help deal with pulmonary aspiration and falling. DVT and PE (lethal blood clots) are most effectively prevented with anticoagulants which come with a completely different set of problems, ranging from longer healing times for cuts and bruises to undue stress on your liver.

Regular blood tests that monitor lipid panels, liver enzymes, hemoglobin, and blood glucose are required. Guys, if your nose bleeds in the winter due to indoor heat drying out your nasal membranes, get used to increased frequency and longer recovery. Check with your primary care Doc to see if you are a viable candidate for an anticoagulant. You may not be. Maybe you're one of the lucky ones with a slow clotting blood chemistry, but if you do need 'em, it's one more pill every day – for the rest of your life.

CHAPTER 7

Battle Campaign

Coping Tactics
Self-Administration of the Heimlich Maneuver
Protective Falling

Coping Tactics[5]

In the IT community when different tasks are contending for the same resource or when a systemic failure programmatically reroutes the process flow to back-up resources, that is known as a "workaround." The following tactics work around dopamine deficiency blockades on the neural pathways to my brain's pattern library when I'm "off my meds."

Swallowing (internally imposed patterns – binary machine language;

internally developed patterns – firmware;

acquired patterns – message transport layer)

Most people don't *THINK* about swallowing. We just do it. Swallowing is a neuromuscular reflex process comprised of conscious, sub-conscious, and autonomic activities. Instigated in the mouth, it is an essential function of digestion. Additionally, swallowing keeps the organs of the mouth and throat moist and lubricated, thereby enabling vocalization and respiration. A moist, throat helps prohibit the ingestion of harmful bacteria.

Since swallowing is a motor function, it is impaired by Parkinson's. Movement of the *epiglottis* (a tissue flap that covers the *trachea* as food and drink pass over it while traversing from the mouth to the *esophagus*) is an autonomic action. PD causes the epiglottis to malfunction and the trachea ingests particles causing pulmonary aspiration (choking).

PD sufferers must concentrate to swallow. Gaping (mouth breathing) is another common symptom. Coupled with not swallowing, it causes the throat to dry, inviting airborne diseases through an open gateway unfiltered by the sinuses. It also leads to other PD mouth-related maladies such as hoarseness

---

5. These sections are neither advisory nor suggestive, but only informational in their content. Although I personally use many of the coping tactics in this book, I do not advise or prescribe their use. If the reader chooses to employ any of these tactics he/she fully understands that any risk associated with doing so is assumed by the reader in making the attempt; and neither the authors, publishers, nor their agents are liable in any form to any degree.

of speech, drooling, and eating problems. The tactic is easy to do and equally easy to forget: swallow every 10 – 15 seconds.

Here's how I take multiple pills. I have a small pill cup, about the size of a *Dixie Cup*® cut in half. I put the pills that I am to take for a single dose into the cup. I drink a little water before I take the pills to lubricate my throat and wake up my epiglottis. I then pour the pills from the cup into my mouth and gulp (swallow forcefully, with vigor) 4 – 6 ounces of water. If you have a method that works better for you, use it. This works for me.

One final note on this topic: among the things that are difficult to swallow are small, dry, uncoated pills. Typical medication dosages may require taking as many as a dozen pills over the course of a day to relieve the symptoms of PD. Two of the most common of these symptoms are loss of manual dexterity (picking up the pills with your fingers) and swallowing these tiny little discs. *Does anyone else find it ironic that the manufacturers of the pills we require are either unaware or don't care that the use of their products is hampered by the symptoms those products are supposed to relieve? Hey! Pharmaceutical companies – NEWS FLASH! Your PD pills hard to grasp and harder to swallow!*

Drooling (internally developed patterns – firmware)
This unsightly embarrassment usually occurs when **a)** you're concentrating on a task requiring manual dexterity (also MIA), **b)** you're looking down at what you're doing; **c)** your mouth is open or your tongue is wagging between your lips; and **d)** you don't swallow. Just because you don't swallow doesn't mean that your salivary glands stop producing liquid inside your mouth. With your head down, your mouth open, and gravity being what it is, the result is inevitable. To avoid drooling, follow these simple steps:

1.   Close your mouth. Lightly lick your lips, then press them together, tightly with the lower lip slightly protruding, for a few seconds to create a moisture seal.

2. Ensure that your teeth are touching – lower to upper, side to side. No need to clench your jaw, just make sure that your teeth are touching.

3. Position of your tongue inside your teeth – not between them or, worse, sticking out between your lips. Many people subconsciously clench their teeth and curl their lips when exerting strength (e.g. opening a jar lid) or stick out their tongues when concentrating on delicate finger play (e.g. tying a fishing lure). Don't do either of these. Keep your tongue in your mouth, and keep your mouth closed.

4. Swallow frequently – at least once every 10 – 15 seconds.

5. Chewing gum is a helpful tactic for all undesired mouth activity; **provided** that you can do so with your mouth closed and *without* biting your tongue.

If you don't already carry a handkerchief, you'll want to start. No matter how careful you are or how many precautions you take, there will still be times when you'll need it.

Blinking (internally imposed patterns – binary machine language)
Before PD, the only times that I thought about blinking was when I either had some foreign debris in my eye or when I was trying to hold back tears. Now, I blink but not as often as I should, and my eyes dry, then they water and burn. The solution is simple. Blink more often. You have to *THINK* about it, though. Add *Blinking* to your *concentration checklist*. Extended periods of intricate hand-eye coordination, TV watching, or video viewing tend to inhibit blinking, drying your eyes that much faster. Be vigilant about frequent, active blinking when engaged in such activities. If your eyes do dry, water, and burn, **_don't_** rub them. Close them and gently blot them with a clean facial tissue. Use your handkerchief only in an emergency. It's not clean. It's been in your pocket, and you've been using it to wipe drool from your chin. If the problem persists, get some eye drops – the ones most like human tears.

Eating (acquired patterns – application layer)
This is a tough one. It involves controlled use of utensils through palsy tremors – cutting with knife and fork, balancing food on a fork or spoon; (twirling
spaghetti onto a fork? *Fagetaboudit.*) opening your mouth without drooling;
inserting a food-laden utensil into your mouth without poking yourself in the
eye; chewing the food sufficiently to swallow without biting your tongue, and
swallowing without choking, coughing, and spitting the entire mouthful across
the table into your boss' face and hair after she so graciously invited you to her
club for a *1-on-1* lunch meeting. Sure – you laugh, but know this: there are only
two kinds of PD sufferers: those who've done it and those who are gonna do it.

This, of course, assumes that the meal is prepared for you. If you think
you're capable of slicing & dicing or sautéing & simmering anything much beyond the standard PD self-prepared lunch (see the next section on *Diet*), have
plenty of *Band-Aids*® and burn ointment readily available, and have someone
standing by to help you apply them.

I avoid utensils, if possible. I prefer food that I can pick up with my
hands – *both* hands during tremors. You can try holding that hot dog in one
hand. Don't worry about the catsup stain on your shirt. Just pre-soak it in cold
water with *OxyClean*®. Take it off, first.

If utensils are unavoidable, do your best to observe proper etiquette, but
quietly and discreetly do whatever you must to get the food into your mouth.
Have a non-alcoholic drink and a napkin ready. Close your mouth. Keep your
tongue in. Swallow frequently.

1. Take small bites. This may be difficult. If your hand is shaking, precise
   utensil loading may be beyond your capabilities.
2. Ask someone to cut the food, if required. In a restaurant, quietly ask
   the server to have your food cut in the kitchen.
3. As much possible, stick with foods that can be stabbed with a fork.
   Don't try to balance foods that can't be stabbed (e.g. peas or salad) on
   a fork. Use a spoon.

4. To scoop food on to your fork, you can use a piece of bread or a roll as a backstop.
5. If you need help from your fingers, that's OK.
6. Swallow before you open your mouth.
7. Insert the utensil with the food. Close your mouth. Remove the utensil.
8. Chew the food thoroughly, then chew it some more. Swallow vigorously.
9. Chase each mouthful with liquid.

Coughing & Choking (internally imposed patterns – binary machine language)

Most of the time, your epiglottis will function properly. When it fails, you'll need your napkin. Go with the cough. Don't try to suppress it or continue to swallow in spite of coughing. Open your mouth, but cover it, and close your teeth to help block any spewing. Your trachea will clear either down into your esophagus, or up into your mouth. If the latter, either discreetly spit the mouthful into your napkin or try re-chewing it into several smaller, morsels. Hold morsels to be re-chewed under your tongue, from where passage into your throat is impossible.

Once your trachea clears, drink liquid after each swallow of food. If you can't clear your trachea enough to breathe, you're choking. **DON'T PANIC**. Get help to perform the *Heimlich Maneuver* on you. If no help is available, you must perform the Heimlich on yourself.

Self-Administration of the Heimlich Maneuver[6]

— Source: wikihow.com

The Heimlich Maneuver is the most common technique used to save a choking person. If no one else is around who is able to assist you, you can save your own life. Follow a few simple steps to learn how to perform the Heimlich Maneuver on yourself.

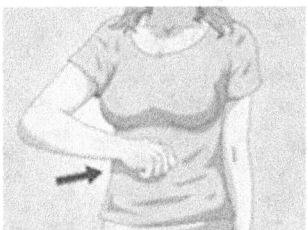

1. ***Make a fist.*** Place it on your abdomen above the navel – just below the ribcage.

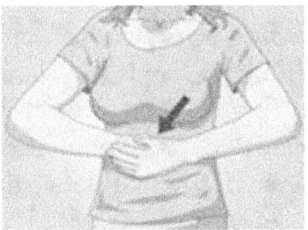

2. ***Hold the fist with your other*** hand for leverage, placing it over the fist, ensuring that it is centered on your stomach. This will allow you to push harder.

---

6. First, check with your physician. Second, seek professional training.

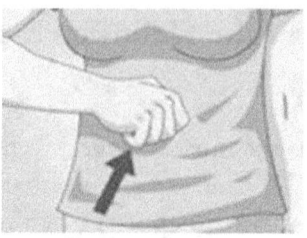

3. ***Drive your fist up into your abdomen.*** Use a quick j-shaped motion, in and up. Repeat. If the debris is not cleared after several attempts, add force with a stable object.

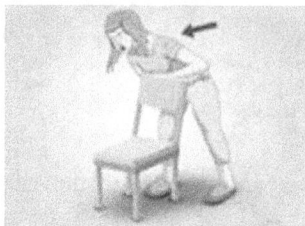

4. ***Add force with a stable object*** that you can bend over – a chair, table, or counter top. With your hands still clasped in front, bend over the object. Brace your fists between your abdomen and the object and drive your body against it. This will increase the force applied to your diaphragm and more effectively dislodge the object.

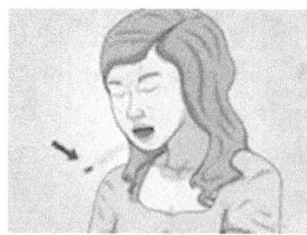

5. ***Repeat.*** If at first you don't succeed – try, try again. Repeat pushing yourself onto the stable object until the obstruction is cleared and you return to normal breathing.

Although you must act quickly and decisively, **DON'T PANIC**. Panicking will only increase your heart rate and need for air, which will make matters worse. Once the obstruction is cleared, sit down. Catch your breath. Seek medical attention for any adverse result.

If all efforts are unsuccessful and before you lose consciousness, ***CALL 9-1-1***.

This is not a procedure that you want to learn during a crisis. Both you and your care giver should learn the Heimlich and the Self-Heimlich. Hold a clean ping-pong ball with your lips (no, don't swallow it), and try to dislodge it with the Heimlich and Self-Heimlich.

Diet (acquired patterns – application layer)
Being afflicted with Parkinson's, you will quickly group food into four categories: (1) food you can taste; (2) food that you like; (3) food that is good for you; and (4) food you can swallow. When you find a food that fits all four categories, stock up.

Standard issue fruits and vegetables will provide the antioxidants that help prevent cell damage – the basis of your affliction. Protein-rich foods like meats, eggs, milk, and peanut butter will kick the *L-DOPA* into gear. There's a theory that caffeine may ease PD symptoms, delaying dementia and being bed-ridden. I am testing a similar theory with ice cream. My preferred Parkinson's lunch is two peanut butter & grape jelly sandwiches chased by a *Mountain Dew*®.

Although alcohol consumption is not prohibited, timing is critical. ***DO NOT*** drink alcohol in any form within 90 minutes prior to or 60 minutes after taking your meds. Otherwise, the alcohol will neutralize the medication. If you do drink alcohol, do so in strict moderation – one glass of beer or wine, three times/week, with twenty-four hours between; *OR* one ounce of hard liquor (> 30% alcohol by volume), twice/week, with forty-eight hours separation. If you have an addiction to alcohol, it's time to seriously consider taking STEP ONE.

Speech (acquired patterns – application layer)
    "Huh?"

    "What?"

    "Pardon me?"

    "Say again?"

You may as well get used to these phrases because you're going to be asked to repeat yourself, often. Your speech will become slurred. You will mumble. You will speak so softly that others will think that you are whispering. Those who don't know you and don't know that you have Parkinson's may take you for being inebriated.

The APDA[7] cites three problems that contribute to speech disorders in Parkinson's: *motor, sensory,* and *cueing.* Motor problems including slow, jerky muscle movement, which are the most obvious sign of Parkinson's disease, affect the diaphragm, larynx and tongue. Parkinson's patients also have sensory processing disorders that make it difficult to hear their voice is getting too soft. Finally, while they are able to respond to external directions to speak louder, they have difficulty cueing the behavior in themselves.

Concentrate on speaking slowly and emphatically, at a volume that may seem offensive. Enunciate clearly. Don't worry about offending your listeners by overemphasizing and oversimplifying what you are saying. Swallow before each time you open your mouth. You don't want drool to distract your audience.

---

7. American Parkinson's Disease Association

Clear your throat, both so that you don't accidentally inhale saliva as you gather breath to speak and to ensure that your larynx is ready for speech. Speak in short, simple sentences. Use words of no more than three syllables, formed clearly and concisely. Inhale with short, shallow breaths. Pause to ensure that your listeners hear you accurately.

Olfactory Sense (autonomic patterns – basic machine language internally developed patterns – firmware)
I don't know if my lost sense of smell is common to PD. It is both good and bad. I am deprived of enjoying pleasant odors but spared enduring foul ones. More importantly, I can't detect dangerous odors (gas leaks, smoke, etc.) and the warnings that they herald. If I ever lose my care giver, Kim, I will get a dog that barks when it smells a dangerous odor. So far, the biggest impact of this impairment is that it weakens taste.

Savory Sense (autonomic patterns – basic machine language internally developed patterns – firmware)
I am not able to distinguish and identify the subtle differences in food flavor. About the only sensation that I am able to experience is how food "feels" in my mouth. Fortunately, I am married to a gourmet chef who prepares food that not only has exotic flavors but also has exotic textures, thereby making the food palatable and the meals interesting.

Balance (internally imposed patterns – binary machine language; internally developed patterns – firmware)
Archimedes of Syracuse was a 2nd Century B.C. Sicilian wise guy. He fiddled with levers, fulcrums, pulleys, cables, and screws; postulated theorems from which, eighteen centuries later, Sir Isaac Newton would develop the *Laws of Gravity* and *Motion*. He liked to holler "*Eureka!*" a lot when he was in the tub. As is often the case with science, man thinks that he has conceived something entirely new only to discover that God already holds a *prior art* patent. The human body's entire skeletal and muscular systems are actually an elegant assembly of levers, fulcrums, pulleys, cables, and screws.

Whachoo tellin' me? Huh? Dat some Sicilian figures he's the first wise guy to use leverage? Hey, Archie – **Fagetaboudit.**

In humans, balance is linked to a physical characteristic common to all solid objects in our universe called the "*center of gravity*." For smaller objects, the center of gravity is equivalent to the physical "*center of mass*." Because space in our Universe is comprised of three dimensions – height, width, and depth – unarticulated solid objects can rotate on any of three axes: longitudinal front-rear rotation, termed *pitch*; horizontal side-side rotation, termed *yaw*; and transverse side-side rotation, termed *roll*.

Here's an "**on meds only**" exercise that will demonstrate human three-dimensional movement. Stand erect with your arms straight out from your shoulders, wing-like. Now, keeping your upper body stiff, lean slightly forward at the waist and return upright. That's *pitch*. Next, upper body still stiff, twist at the waist, clockwise then counter-clockwise, keeping your arms parallel to the ground. That's *yaw*. Finally, rock sideways at the waist, first right – then left. That's *roll*. Combining maneuvers results in the body's full range of motions. Don't get cocky. Cartwheels are no longer in your repertoire.

The human body has many articulated joints. Ankles, knees, hips, shoulders, and the spinal vertebrae are primary, regarding balance. The body's center of gravity repositions with changes in physical attitude (lying, standing, sitting) and posture. Add the physical phenomena *momentum* and *inertia*, impacting a body in *motion*, and you get an idea of the complex patterns required to move your body while balancing it on two feet.

Balance is the human brain's combined visual-aural-tactile sensory perception. Through autonomic focusing of their stereoscopic vision, the eyes act like a carpenter's level, and the middle ear *Eustachian Tubes* equalize differences in atmospheric pressure.

"Sensory information about motion, equilibrium, and spatial orientation is provided by the VESTIBULAR *apparatus in each ear, which includes the* UTRICLE, SACCULE, *and three* SEMICIRCULAR CANALS. *The utricle and saccule detect gravity (vertical orientation) and linear movement. The semicircular canals detect rotational movement. Located at right angles to each other, they are filled with the fluid,* ENDOLYMPH."[8]

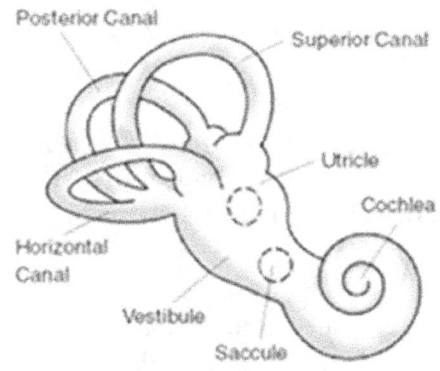

SOURCE: Web-Books.com

The vestibular system senses *motion, momentum,* and *inertia* and responds with sophisticated reflexes to stabilize the head and body while compensating for the Earth's gravitational attraction. The three semicircular canals influence the three axes of motion around the body's Center of Gravity. The *horizontal canal* regulates motion along the *yaw axis, while the superior* and *posterior canals* join forces to regulate motion along both the *pitch* and *roll axes.*

Electromagnetic conductors engage the assembled neural, muscular, and skeletal systems' levers, fulcrums, cables, and pulleys to orchestrate the body's movements. The three senses collaborate to access recognized patterns to keep the head perched atop the neck, the neck atop the torso, the torso atop the legs, and the whole structure balanced on two feet as they move the body about the planet's surface. Human mobility patterns are deeply imbedded in the pattern library somewhere between the subconscious and the autonomic user interfaces.

Children often play at making themselves dizzy, disrupting their balance perception by rapidly spinning in circles until they fall down. Parkinson's sufferers don't play at falling. Since stereoscopic focus, posture control, gaze stability, and mobility are muscle controlled activities, their dysfunction and

---

8. The *Vestibular Disorders Association* – http://vestibular.org/understanding-vestibular-disorder/human-balance-system

resulting falls due to loss of balance is a common PD symptom, as is the absence of counter-balancing arm-swing in a PD sufferer's gait.

"*Good to know*" you say, "*but how does knowing all of this* (Have you ever met anyone with so much useless noise in his head? O – m'G! He's the Cliff Clavin of Parkinson's! Blah, blah, blah!) *help me to walk across the room without falling on my ass?*"

OK, fair question. First tip (sorry for the pun) – figure skaters and dining room servers. Remember the spinning children? A spinning figure skater doesn't allow her head to spin with her body, but she turns her head separately from her body and momentarily locks her focus on fixed objects within her rotating field of vision. Likewise, a server balancing a tray of food on one hand held above his head never looks at the tray. He focuses on some fixed object beyond his destination table but in line with his intended path to that table. So when walking, actively focus on a target object across the room, across the yard, down the sidewalk, or wherever along your intended line of travel; frequently glancing down to check for trippers.

Next tip – rock climbing. Nope. Never done it. Don't want to do it. Afraid of heights. There is, however, a rock climbing axiom that is useful to PD sufferers: "*Always maintain three points of contact with the rock face.*" In other words, of a climber's two hands + two feet, three of the four appendages should be in contact with the rock face at all times, while the fourth is purchasing a new handhold or foothold. In short, when standing or walking with PD, hang on to something – a staircase railing, a chair, a cane, or a walker. What? Too proud to use a cane or a walker? How proud are you when you fall on your coccyx in the parking lot at *Walmart*®?

You also have a fifth point of contact not available to rock climbers – your butt. Give up trying to do things while standing that can be done just as easily – easier, in fact – while seated (e.g. putting your pants on, one leg at-a-time). Sit down before you fall down.

Final tip – when standing, position your feet at shoulder-width slightly offset, front-to-rear. Distribute your weight along the length of your foot. The balls of your feet are the fulcrums upon which your legs are levered. Your heels prevent *pitching* to the rear and falling. Think of them as "training heels." This four-point base is your foundation. Your center of gravity is in your butt. Ensure that it is squarely centered on that base – back straight, shoulders back and parallel to the ground, head up, eyes focused (hey – CLOSE YOUR MOUTH – SWALLOW – BLINK). Don't lock your knees. Bend them slightly for leverage to help your eyes, ears, muscles, tendons, and neural transmitters balance the load.

After standing for several minutes, you may feel dizzy. You are about to fall. Avoid stumbling in the direction of the fall trying to regain your balance. You'll only add momentum to the fall and increase its severity. Instead, grab a stable object. If no stable anchor is within reach, try to find some place to sit – the floor, if necessary. A sudden, ungraceful plop on your butt is embarrassing, but it's better than falling backward through a plate glass door.

More help is offered in the following sections of this book: *Posture, Mobility, Walking, Sitting Down & Arising, Lying Down & Arising, Preventing Falls, Protective Reactions When Falling, Recovering From a Fall,* and *Changing Positions in Bed.*

Posture (acquired patterns – application layer)
It is important that you maintain as vertically straight a posture in your spine as you can. Parkinson's sufferers tend to hump their shoulders when standing and "list" to one side when seated. For most people, the human body's center of gravity is in the butt. Whether sitting or standing, keep your shoulders squarely parallel to the ground and your head vertically aligned straight above your butt. Obviously, lying down has different rules.

Mobility (acquired patterns – application layer)
Moving the body applies the mechanics of motion, momentum, and inertia through the use of levers, fulcrums, cables, pulleys, and screws; all countered by gravity and electromagnetism. Sounds simple enough, but try to imagine how many muscle memory patterns that I accessed just in typing this one paragraph composed of 55 words with 348 characters.

Animal mobility is truly a miracle of the universe, and the entire animal kingdom benefits from that miracle. While our bodies are still forming in the womb, we learn to move. Once out of the womb, we begin the process of learning and mastering bi-pedal ambulation. As our bodies develop, we add mobility skills: running, dancing, throwing, swimming. When we move, we don't consciously expand and contract muscles or articulate joints. We just do it. Well, "we" don't just do it, anymore. "We" have Parkinson's disease. "We" must *THINK* about moving before "we" can *actually* move. Our "*re*" has no "*flex*."

Walking (acquired patterns – application layer)
Anyone who has endured military boot camp has been thoroughly drilled in the *Manuel of Arms*. Among other things, they learned how to salute, how to handle a rifle, and how to march. LEFT – RIGHT. LEFT – RIGHT, lock stepping in a straight line, eyes forward, backs straight, the only movement above the waist is the counter-balancing arm swing with each step, guide-on at the point, pennants streaming below the Star Spangled Banner hoisted high. There is nothing quite so stirring as a cadre of warriors on parade. The basics of marching are found in the mechanics of walking, so let's re-learn how to walk by reverse-engineering the process of marching. *Ten-HUT!*

That's right. We're starting with our upright stance – feet firmly planted at shoulder-width and slightly offset front-to-rear; spine comfortably straight with shoulders back and parallel to the ground; arms hanging loosely from the shoulders; head up with eyes focused and knees slightly bent. Now, CLOSE YOUR MOUTH –SWALLOW – BLINK.

1. Lift your left foot. I know – your brain wants to slide it forward. Concentrate. Lift your left foot – not high – a couple of inches. This is the most important task in walking. You must constantly remember to pick up your feet. Don't shuffle them.
2. As you're doing that, pitch (remember pitch?) your upper body slightly forward, shifting your weight to the ball of your right foot by slightly raising your right heel.

3. Extend your left leg forward from the knee, using your body's pitch momentum.

4. Plant your left heel ahead of your right foot, shifting your weight to your left heel.

5. Lift your right foot. Extend it forward. Shift your weight to the ball of your left foot.

6. Plant your right heel ahead of your left foot and shift your weight to it.

7. *Success!* You have walked two steps – one pace – forward.

8. Now, repeat the process but this time, take four steps = two paces.

9. Eight steps = four paces.

10. Continue without stopping.

11. Add arm-swing; i.e. loosely relax your right arm and swing it forward simultaneously with moving your left leg forward and vice-versa – left arm, right leg. This counter-balances your body's weight distribution while it is momentarily perched on one leg. Arm-swing is essential to human bi-pedal ambulation (walking, running, dancing, etc.) It is such a natural motion, that we do it without thinking (again, the generic "we" – people not suffering from Parkinson's). Competitive runners are taught to coordinate arm-swing with leg-stride. Distance runners keep their lower arms parallel to the ground, driving them like pistons, back-and-forth, straight in their direction of travel. Sprinters cock their lower arms in an upward angle to quicken their pace. Longer arm-swing = longer leg-stride. Faster arm-swing = faster pace. When you're having trouble getting the required momentum to take that first step, consciously swing your arm as you lift your opposing leg.

12. Try turning. Turn right by pivoting on the ball of your left foot. Turn left by pivoting on the ball of your right foot. Turn around by pivoting twice in the same direction.

13. **NEVER WALK BACKWARD.** Your balance can no longer manage such a complex move. Better to turn around and prevent a serious head injury resulting from a fall.

True, you've been doing this without thinking since before your 1st birthday. When meds are ON, it will be as easy as ever, but when meds are OFF, *THINKing* will be required.

Sitting Down & Arising (acquired patterns – application layer)
Probably the first thing you learned after taking your first step was how to sit.
No – that's not correct. After taking that first step, you probably learned how
to fall. If that fall after your first step landed on your butt, Mom and Dad
probably tagged it as "learned to sit."

The process hasn't changed from that first plop. Your center of gravity is
still near your butt. Start by pitching your entire body slightly backward from
the ankles. Then simultaneously lever your upper legs down at the knees and
lever your upper body forward at the hips, positioning your center of gravity,
vertically, over the balls of your feet.

You will find that you prefer armchairs The chair arms provide the fulcrums upon which your articulated arm levers lower your center-of-gravity
butt into and hoist it out of a seated position. *Fair warning*: avoid seats that
don't have something to grip for stability.

To stand from a seated position, grip the arms of the chair tightly with
both hands. Close your mouth – swallow – blink. With your butt as close to
the edge as you can get it without sliding off and with the balls of your feet
as near to vertically aligned with your center of gravity as you can get, *pitch*
forward until all of your weight is on your legs and feet. Finally, straighten you
knees and your hips into an upright position.

Lying Down & Arising (acquired patterns – application layer)
Getting into bed when you are adequately medicated is so much easier than when
you're not. There are all the preparations – nighttime ablutions, changing into
sleepwear, turning down the bed covers, turning out the lights. Then you must
climb into bed, pull the covers up, and get into a comfortable position for sleeping.

You don't want to attempt all of this when you're off your meds. You'll be
so worn out that you won't be able to sleep. If you are off your meds, ask your
care giver for help with changing into sleepwear and getting into bed. For one
night give yourself permission to forego the ablutions. If you are alone, you
can always just grab a blanket, crash into a recliner, and sleep in your street

clothes, however, there will be a price to pay in the morning (see the sections on *Changing Positions in Bed* and *Sleeping*).

The ease or difficulty with which you are able to get out of bed will depend on the quality of sleep you experienced overnight. Six to eight hours of uninterrupted, deep sleep goes a long way in enabling the motor skills required to transition from lying horizontally to standing vertically. First, get entirely out from under the covers. Your lower body is already encumbered – you don't need to get your feet tangled in the sheets. Next, raise both your head and your feet slightly and pivot your body on your butt 90° until your legs extend out of the bed, perpendicular to the side of the mattress. Grip the edge of the mattress tightly. *Pitch* your body forward and use the momentum of your lower body reaching the floor to help your arms pull your upper body into a sitting position on the side of the bed. CLOSE YOUR MOUTH – SWALLOW – BLINK. With your butt on the edge of the bed and with the balls of your feet vertically aligned with your center of gravity, *pitch* forward. When all your weight is on your feet, stand up.

Sleeping (internally developed patterns – firmware)
A good night's sleep is worth ¼ of a dose of meds. 7 – 8 solid sleeping hours starting between 9:00 & 10:00 P M gives muscle control to get my day started with a minimum of PD symptom interference and may last as long as an hour. That's enough time for me to get out of bed, go to the bathroom, and fix a protein shake to drink with my first round of meds. 20 – 30 minutes later, they kick in, and I'm ready for my A.M. routine: exercise, morning ablutions, grooming, and dressing – all by myself, like a big boy and everything. The day starts well, and days that start well usually go well.

I know. You want to stay up to watch the 11:00 PM (E)/10:00 PM (C) news and the late night talk shows. Trust me. Just DVR 'em. You can watch 'em the next day and fast-forward through all those PIA pharmaceutical commercials and whatever other superfluous crap that you prefer to do without. You watch too much TV, anyway.

An earlier bedtime means that you will be getting ready for and into bed while that day's last round of meds is still in play. Again, all of that is much easier without the extracurricular shaking, fumbling, stumbling, and drooling distractions. Make sure that you include a trip to the toilet. After the meds go down, there's no such thing as a quick response to an urgent, middle-of-the-night pee call.

For bedding, you'll want to avoid heavy comforters, quilts, and blankets. As you'll see in the next section, heavy bedding makes changing position that much more difficult later, when the meds do wear off. During warm weather, I cover with only a sheet. When it's cold, I add a light thermal blanket topped by a light micro-weave fleece blanket. Cozy.

For Summer sleepwear, I prefer boxers – modest coverage that's loose enough to be comfortable, but not so long as to tangle my feet and make changing position all the more difficult. In the Winter, I add a thinly woven, snug-fitting, long-sleeved T-shirt (no buttons) for upper body warmth and socks to keep my feet warm.

I used to sleep on my stomach. That stopped with the neck surgery in 2002. The neurosurgeon said the way I positioned my head when sleeping on my stomach contributed to the herniated disc. Now, I sleep on either side or flat on my back. With Parkinson's I've had to reposition my right arm to quiet the tremors. When I lie on my right side, I jam my open right hand (palm up) under the pillow, directly beneath my right ear. Lying on my left side, I clench my right hand between my thighs. When lying on my back, I jam my open right hand (palm up) under my right thigh. Again, these positions work for me. You'll have to find your own adaptations. Whatever it takes to get as much relaxed, restful sleep as you can. You'll need it.

Changing Position in Bed (acquired patterns – application layer)
There's no secret sauce for this one. It's just plain difficult. Usually, by the time the middle of the night rolls around and you need to change position, your meds will have worn off. You have no idea the extent of controlled muscle coordination required to execute this maneuver until you have to do it in an uncontrollable state.

If you like to sleep on your stomach, get over it. Those nights are gone. I will describe switching from lying on one side to lying on the other. If you want to start from or stop at lying on your back, that's the halfway point in the move. Sleeping on your side –

1. "Top" is your body's "up" side, and "bottom" is the side upon which you are lying.
2. Disentangle the covers and use your top hand to hold them out of the way.
3. Fold your legs at the knees into a semi-fetal position.
4. With your bottom hip and elbow as fulcrums and using your bottom leg and arm as levers, roll your body onto your back and sit up.
5. Switch hands holding the covers.
6. Now, the two sides are reversed – i.e. "top" becomes "bottom" and vice-versa.
7. Roll toward your target bottom side, reversing the lever/fulcrum process of your bottom arm/leg and elbow/hip. Scooch in any final adjustments that you need.
8. Go back to sleep.

This maneuver requires practice without which, you will struggle through it to the point of such exhaustion that you won't be able to sleep. Worse – you'll probably disturb your partner to the point that *she* won't be able to sleep. Keep peace in the bed – practice.

Protective Falling

80,000 – 100,000 people who suffer from Parkinson's disease die each year from fatal complications related to the disease. The majority of these fatalities are the result of falls. Sufferers can employ these protective measures to reduce the risk and impact of falling, but the unfortunate reality is that the disorder blocks the neural pathways from accessing the afflicted brain's balance patterns that are required to stand erect, unassisted, a circumstance over which sufferers have no control and thus, no protection.

Fall Prevention (acquired patterns – application layer)
Preventing falls basically comes down to situational awareness – surroundings, surface, motion preparation, proper balance, and judgement. In addition to the previously de-scribed focal point concentration and "three points of con-tact," follow some simple rules.

1. Wear shoes with non-slip soles – no flip-flops. Avoid slippery surfaces.
2. Look around your feet. Ensure that there are no obstacles that might trip you.
3. Avoid long, flowing floor-length clothing.
4. Walk – don't run. Swing your arms to counter-balance moving your legs.
5. Concentrate on maintaining your balance. Lean slightly forward, keeping your center of gravity vertically aligned over the balls of your feet.
6. Pick up your feet. Don't shuffle them.
7. If you feel you're losing your balance, grab hold of something. Sit down, if necessary. Don't be too embarrassed to ask for help.
8. Don't try to balance on one leg while pulling on pants, overshoes, etc.
9. Always be aware of your balance. Don't lean so far in any one direc-tion so that your balance becomes unrecoverable.
10. Stay off ladders – avoid climbing.
11. When negotiating stairs, use the handrail. Lean slightly backward go-ing downstairs and slightly forward going upstairs. That way if you do fall, you'll fall in a direction opposite to the incline and will be less likely to suffer serious injury. *NEVER* carry anything requiring both hands while going up or down stairs. If your view is obscured, count the stair-step risers as you climb or descend. Standard staircases typi-cally have fourteen risers, but not all staircases are standard, so hang on to the handrail.
12. Don't carry heavy, difficult-to-balance, or large bulky objects that ob-scure your view.
13. Always have your emergency communications device with you if you need help.
14. At some point, you'll need a walker. Better to get it too soon rather than too late.

Protective Reactions When Falling (acquired patterns – application layer)
Defensive driving tactics anticipate danger and have a contingency plan to escape, if the danger materializes. Single-engine aircraft pilots constantly look for suitable emergency landing fields, in the event of engine failure. So should you always be thinking, while in motion, about where and how you can land if you fall. On what kind of surface are you standing (assume falling from a standing position – falls while sitting or lying down are so rare)? Is there a softer surface nearby? What dangerous obstacles, particularly, what glass objects are in range? What can you grab to help prevent a fall? What help can you summon? Is your emergency communication device immediately at hand? The answers to these questions are all part of being aware of your surroundings.

When you feel yourself starting to fall[9] –

1. **DON'T PANIC.**
2. Try to regain your balance. If you are unable to do that and you're going to fall, you need to try to control the fall so as to minimize injury.
3. Concentrate on relaxing your body. Tense muscles increase the severity of injury. Try to exhale as you fall to help you relax.
4. Protect your head. The most important body part that you need to protect in a fall is your head. Head injuries can be very serious, even fatal. Make sure you prioritize protecting your head as you fall by properly positioning it.
5. Tuck your chin down, lowering your head.
6. If falling backward, crumple at your knees and at your waist. Try to land on your butt in a sitting position.
7. If falling face first, turn your head to the side.
8. Bring your arms up to protect your head – in front of your head if falling forward or behind your head if falling backward. Head injuries include skull fractures, concussions, and brain hemorrhages, all of which are life threatening.

---

9. First, check with your physician. Second: seek professional training.

9. Turn as you fall. If you are falling either straight forward or straight backwards, try to turn your body so you land on your side. Falling directly on your back can cause serious injury. A frontal fall can cause damage to the head, face, and arms. By landing on your side you can reduce the chance of injury.

10. Keep your elbows and knees bent. It's tempting to try and catch yourself as you fall fully with your arms. However, landing with your arms straight out and absorbing the full force of the fall can cause injury. Keeping both your elbows and knees slightly bent as you fall protects your wrists, arms, and shoulders.

11. Roll with the impact. If you're able, spread the force of the fall – roll into it. Transfer the energy of the fall to the roll, rather than taking the impact with your body.

This technique requires practice. Check with your Doc to get medical clearance and a referral to a Licensed Physical Therapist for supervised training and practice on padded, cushioned floors. You may want to consider wearing a helmet and pads on your knees, wrists, and elbows during the training sessions.

Recovering From a Fall (acquired patterns – application layer)

Again, DON'T PANIC. Lie still. Give yourself time to gather your senses. Gently move your extremities to check for injuries. If you are injured or if you were unconscious for any period of time, stay down and activate your emergency communications device. If you are uninjured and did not lose consciousness, carefully try getting to your feet.

1. If face down, roll onto your back using the maneuvers described in the section titled *Changing Position in Bed*. Rest a moment while you check for injuries.

2. Once on your back, carefully raise your upper body into a sitting position. This may require leverage, at first with your elbows, then with your hands.

3. Gently turn your head from side to side. Check that your neck isn't injured and wait for any dizziness to clear.

4. If there is a solidly anchored object within reach, *very carefully* use it to pull yourself to your feet. If nothing is in reach, carefully roll onto your hands and knees.

Method A.

5. With your hands flat on the palms placed wider than your shoulders and your knees together, shift your lower body weight from your knees to the balls of your feet by bending your knees and pitching your upper slightly backward, distributing your weight between the palms of your hands and the balls of your feet.

6. Carefully "walk" your hands backwards toward your feet. This maneuver should, with little effort on your part, shift your upper body weight from your hands to the balls of your feet. Your entire weight is on the balls of your feet. Your arms still reach the ground in front, but that is intended more to keep you from *pitching* too far forward as you execute the next maneuver than it is to bear your weight.

7. As you *pitch* back slightly, shifting your weight from the balls of your feet to fully on both feet (balls-arches-heels), simultaneously raise your upper body at your hips while straightening your knees and ankles. If it helps, steady your upper body by placing your hands on your knees and/or thighs. Once you reach your full, upright position, conduct one last check for injuries and dizziness before you toddle off.

Method B.

5. Raise your upper body to an upright position while "standing" on your knees. Pause to check for injuries and dizziness.

6. Carefully lift one leg and plant its foot firmly on the surface. Place the palms of your hands, one on top of the other on the knee of the planted leg.

7. Using your arms as levers and the knee of your planted leg as a fulcrum, lever your body upward by pushing with your arms while straightening your elbows. When you've raised high enough, plant your other leg and stand erect. Again, give yourself time to check for injuries and stability. — *Source: wikihow.com*

Some people prefer **METHOD B** because they feel it's more graceful. I guess they don't think that **A** is all that flattering. Personally, I prefer **METHOD A** because it's more stable. To each his own. After the **METHOD B**s take a couple of extra falls while trying to get up, they'll worry less about grace. Either way, falls are serious and can be fatal. If you are the least bit concerned about any effects of a fall – seek immediate medical attention.

Handwriting (acquired patterns – application layer)
In the one-room, country school I attended, we had ***penmanship*** contests. I was usually the winning boy in my grade – probably because I was the <u>only</u> boy in my grade. Nevertheless, I always took pride in my handwriting. Kids today don't even learn cursive penmanship. Where will we find the ***Thomas Jeffersons*** and ***James Madisons*** of tomorrow? "Text" is now a verb? O – M'G! The utter travesty of it! I guess I'll just put my fountain pen on the shelf next to my slide rule and analog watch. They're no good, anymore, either. One only calculates complex math problems, and the other only tells time.

Good news – bad news. The bad news is that with Parkinson's, your handwriting, at best, sucks; at worst, it's completely illegible. The good news is – you no longer need it. With all this electronic communication media, no one ***writes*** *anything*. Well, almost no one. I still write one check every three weeks – to my barber. That's right, folks. I found the one barber in America who doesn't take plastic, but I still don't write the check. He fills it out, and I sign it. The bank clears it, even with my lame scribble of a signature.

If possible, avoid handwriting. Embrace the electronic media – "text," e-mail, word processor, portable document format, whatever. You can attach your electronic signature to documents. You can transmit your electronic signature between devices to be attached to a document. The demise of written signatures is fast approaching, to be replaced by biometric devices – fingerprint readers, retina scanners, DNA analyzers, et al. If handwritten media are unavoidable, take your time and use block print characters.

Keyboarding (acquired patterns – application layer)

I have described my keyboarding history. When on the meds, the keyboard is the user friendly tool that it has always been. Without the meds, it's a one-handed nemesis.

Dictation software is some help (if speech is intelligible), but speaking every punctuation mark and paragraph disrupts my flow, and I lose my thoughts. I've tried straight dictation, then adding the punctuation, but that takes more time. No easy answer here.

Short-Term Memory (autonomic patterns – basic machine language)

"The memory is the second thing to go."

"Oh, yeah? What's the first."

"I don't know. I can't remember."

No fool-proof solution here, either. When in a conversation or making a presentation, I will suddenly have to stop, awkwardly gaping while I desperately try to find my words. The pause becomes unbearable. If I don't explain my difficulty to my listeners, someone will offer suggestions in an attempt to help me complete my thought. Someone else will misinterpret my pause as a sign for them to comment. At that point, not only can't I find my words, but also I have forgotten the original topic. Typically, frustration ensues.

Used to be that when I wanted to remember something, I would write it down. Now, I have *two* problems. (1) I can't remember, and (2) I can't read what I wrote. I tried "texting" reminders into my "smart" phone's notepad using the on-screen keyboard with mmuchh the sssamee rressultt as wwithh mmyy ddeskkttopp kkeyybboardd. Next, I tried recording voice notes into my "smart" phone. Slurred speech yielded this result –

Record: *"There's a bad moon out tonight."*
Playback: *"There's a bathroom on the right."*

I tried the speech-to-text feature on my "smart" (*They really aren't, you know. I liked 'em better when they were just phones.*) phone. Same slurred speech, similar result —

Speech: "*I fought the Law, and the Law won.*"
Text: "*I thought her bra was undone.*"

"*Oh, never mind. Just forget it.*"

"*Forget what?*"

"*I don't know.* **I CAN'T REMEMBER!** "

Tremors (internally imposed patterns – basic machine language)
For me, this is the most embarrassing PD symptom — even more so than drooling. As I have described, my lower right arm is most affected by the palsy tremors at a frequency of about three cycles per second. Being right-handed, I can forget about anything as simple as a two seam grip on a baseball, let alone throwing a slider.

If I'm in a conversation or speaking to an audience, the tremors are an unnecessary distraction. It's so pitiful saying, "*Please excuse my right arm. I have Parkinson's.*" I prefer, "*Please excuse my right arm. It thinks that it's the tail of a Golden Retriever, and he's really excited to see you.*" Handshakes become uncontrollable '60s cultural greeting rituals.

If I don't consciously force my arm down to the side of my leg, my hand will come to rest of its own accord in front of my lower abdomen and appear to be miming an obscene gesture (oh, come on – use your imagination). "Hands-on" activities are out of the question: eating, fishing, handwriting, tttyyyypppiinngg, driving, the TV remote. I can clear a chessboard with one move of N – KB3. Shaving? Not just a job – an adventure! One piece of good news – after doing it wrong since I was a child, I'm finally brushing my teeth with the up-and-down motion about which dentists have been scolding me twice a year, for my entire life.

One would think that a simple solution would be to train my left hand to become more dominant. Not so simple, Simon. Using my left hand to do something that I normally would use my right hand to do only makes my right arm tremble more severely. It's like my right arm throws a temper fit, saying "Hey! That's my job. Mind your own business." To which my left arm responds by trembling – kowtowing to the right arm bully. The only means I have found to counteract palsy tremors is to take the medication.

Countenance (autonomic patterns – basic machine language)

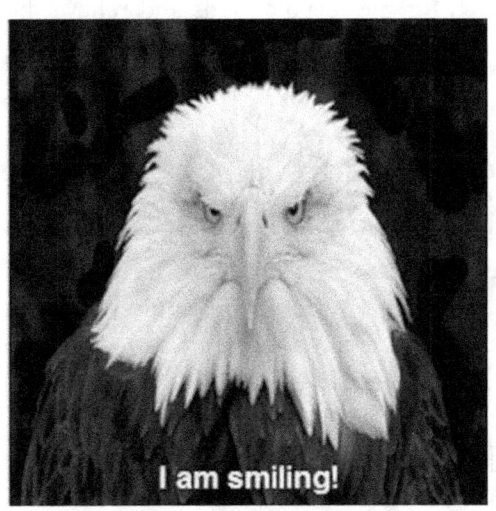

I am smiling!

It's called the *"Parkinson's Mask."* Your face can easily be taken PoW by your brain, if you let your guard down. Everyone will think that you are angry. You may be but most of the time, you'll be perfectly happy, or at worst, just calmly and quietly *THINK*ing; concentrating on something known only to you. This reverie will be innocently disturbed by some kind-hearted soul, *"What's the matter? Now – what is it?"* The "off meds" tactic is vigilant self-awareness. Add another word to your mantra: PICK UP YOUR FEET – SWING YOUR ARMS – CLOSE YOUR MOUTH – SWALLOW – BLINK – *SMILE*.

Manual Dexterity (acquired patterns – application layer)

The opposable thumb is overrated. When you're "off your meds," it often doesn't work. It's just a fifth finger that sticks out to the side and is too short to be of any use. Occupational therapists will have you practice picking up small coins and buttons. Doesn't help. You'll find yourself using both hands to pick up a dime. It will take you three minutes to pull your wallet out of your pocket and get out your debit card. Again, be vigilant, be aware, be prepared – most importantly – stay on your meds.

Muscle Cramps (autonomic patterns – basic machine language)
It has always been my understanding that the Potassium in bananas is supposed to help prevent cramps. I expected my Potassium Chloride/Lasix cocktail would provide a similar benefit. Wrong. Every time that I get behind in my PD medications, the toes of my left foot cramp and curl into a fist. No amount of massaging or will power relieves the club foot that results. I have to get down on my hands and knees and crawl in order to move. Odd, crawling a few feet eases the cramp long enough for me to take meds and relieve the cramp for the day. If I keep up with my meds, this problem is a "no-show."

Driving (acquired patterns – application layer)
Dude (or Dudette) – three words: **ON MEDS ONLY**! College Football Hall of Fame Coach Darrell Royal of the University of Texas Longhorns is generally attributed with saying "*Three things can happen with a forward pass, and two of them are bad.*" Well, I can think of about a dozen things that could happen if anyone with PD would operate a motor vehicle in an unmedicated state, and **ALL** of them are bad. Of course, there may be emergencies. That is what your support network is for – including your mobile emergency contact device. If you find yourself in a life-threatening situation, **CALL 9-1-1**. If no threat exists, but you urgently need transportation when off your meds, call a friend, relative, or neighbor. Worst case – call a taxi or *Uber*. Arrange all of this in your support network.

Driving while physically impaired can easily result in a fatal accident that takes your life or that of another. The least consequential, non-injury circumstance would be one where you are pulled over by law enforcement on suspicion of DUI because you were driving erratically. Sure, you can play the "Parkinson's card" all you want, but your slurred speech and stumbling gait won't help your case in trying to pass a roadside sobriety test. You'll give the cops no choice but to haul you in to donate blood and urine samples – which will, of course, prove that you're not drunk – just stupid. The damage will have been done, however. Most states have *DWI – Driving While Impaired* – laws which expand the DUI laws to include improper use of illicit drugs and failure to take medication required to safely operate a motor vehicle. At that point, both your negligence and your disability are subject to review by a court of law. The court can require that you submit to physical and driving examinations to determine whether your driving privilege should be restricted or revoked – *permanently*.

Now, was that trip to the mall really *that* important. Dude – three words: *ON MEDS ONLY*!

Recreation (acquired patterns – application layer)
I **loved** being a baseball umpire. Spent more than 40 Springs and Summers chasing people ⅓ my age around "*yards*" in five states. Broke my heart when I had to give it up. So many stories – but those are for another book – maybe. Point is, I was passionate about umpiring baseball – never got tired of it. Even wrote a poem about it.

Summer Time Blues

Adrenaline highs, and kick-the-call lows –
A coach in your face; his toes to your toes.
Locker room antics and insider jokes –
Starch, polish, and game face outside for the folks.
See the ball, make the call, take the heat, but don't show it.
They whine and they cry, but it's fair and they know it.
Their tempers get short. Their words get unlawful.
Concession-stand food:
"More filling!"   Tastes awful!"

Sometimes it hurts. You want to say, "Screw it!"
Somebody asks, "Why do you do it?"
You can't find the answer. It's vague and unclear,
But when Spring hits the ball yard, you're back there each year.
You don't know the reason. You're different – that's all –
With this uncanny urge to holler, "PLAY BALL!"
You've got an affliction you're not going to lose.
'Cause "...there ain't no cure for the
                    Summer Time Blues."

With the arrival of Parkinson's, I've had to find a new passion. Thanks to the patient understanding of my friends and family, I have rediscovered fishing. As a boy my step-fathers (yes, I had more than one – another story; another time) taught me to hunt and fish. After Viet Nam, hunting kinda lost its charm. I tried it a couple of times when I came home – no joy. Besides, I was into being a baseball umpire. There was no time to fish.

I don't know if my dear wife really enjoys fishing as much I do. If she doesn't, she doesn't let it show. We have a bass boat and an RV camper. We go camping and fishing almost every weekend in the Spring and Summer. We bought enough fishing and boating gear for a small navy. We have *Cabela's* and *Bass Pro Shops* on speed dial.

During the Summer, we attend at least one outdoor concert a week, and in the Fall, we have season tickets to the Nebraska Cornhusker football games. Driving the RV to the home games, we are serious tailgaters. Through the late Fall and Winter months we entertain in our home. We invite friends to join us for away Husker football games, wine & single-malt tastings, and dinner parties. We have a Holiday Open House every December. We stay engaged with our friends – caring friends who understand that Parkinson's is part of our life and therefore, they willingly make it part of theirs.

"*Engaged.*" That's the key. Parkinson's sufferers must stay actively *engaged* with life. Get out of the chair. Get out of the house. Time your medication doses to enable you to enjoy the best part of each day. Do stuff that interests you. Find fun. Converse. Discuss. Debate. Share. If you're embarrassed or afraid to be with other people, your brain wins.

Employment (acquired patterns – application layer)
You'll want to keep working as long as you can. There will be some vocations that will eliminate themselves. Concert Pianist, Neurosurgeon, Court Reporter, and Explosive Ordinance Disposal Technician come immediately to mind, but there are many others. You may not be able to continue with your chosen career, but in the interest of staying mentally and physically active, you

need to do something. A steady source of income is always welcome, plus you feel better about yourself if you can contribute to your own well-being and to the well-being of those you love. If you have worked a long time in your career, you have expertise to offer on a consulting basis. Modern communications have simplified working from home.

This, too, will require strict medication timing. Be fair to your employer and advise them that there may be an unfavorable impact resulting from your employment. Tasks assigned to you may require more time to complete than if they were assigned to able-bodied workers. There may be some extraordinary expense associated with specialized hardware, software, communication, access, etc. The company's healthcare insurance premiums may increase. Consider working part-time so as not to affect the cost of healthcare benefits for other employees.

You may be of more value to your employer than employees with less experience, but you may cost more in terms of task completion time and the extra support that you require. Keep these factors in mind when negotiating your compensation package.

Dressing (acquired patterns – application layer)
Ladies, this is one of those gender related areas that I mentioned earlier. I'm sorry – I can't advise you, in this regard. I am a man. Sure, I figured out how to unsnap a bra with two fingers when I was sixteen, but I wouldn't have the first clue about how to hook one in place, behind my back, with my shaking hands, and my dysfunctional manual dexterity.

Lifelong friends like buttons, zippers, and shoelaces are, now, hated enemies. You will find that the more you can avoid them, the easier life will be. Wear "low maintenance" clothing: shirts without buttons, shoes without laces, and no neckties. Think "*Velcro*®."

After you decide what to wear, you have get dressed. If ever there was a "keep it simple" justification for your daily routine, it's dressing with Parkinson's. As I mentioned earlier, this task is **_so_** much easier after you have taken your medication. Do as much as possible while seated. Don't try to put on underwear and pants while standing. That's a certain fall. Doing more while sitting will be one of your biggest changes. After you pull your pants on, lying back on the bed makes buttoning them and tightening your belt easier. Of course then you're faced with the whole *Stand Up From Lying Down* thing.

Bathing (acquired patterns – application layer)
First question: "*Tub or shower?*" Falls can happen entering or exiting either. My balance is still pretty good, so I prefer the shower. That's how I've bathed my whole life. The shower doors are glass, though, and I worry about falling with enough force to break them and suffering a catastrophic accident. Like everything else I do these days, I make sure that I've taken my meds, and I concentrate as much as I can on what I am doing. If I do decide to take a bath, I use the built-in seat to ease myself fully into the tub.

I haven't noticed any change due to PD in my bathing routine. Soap, water, shampoo, washcloth, drying towel – all pretty much work as before. I shave in the shower. Remember? "*Not just a job – an adventure!*" Water is immediately available to wash away the blood. Never more the case than with PD. Take your meds – less hemorrhaging.

Grooming (acquired patterns – application layer)
I've discussed shaving and teeth brushing. If you're so inclined, electric appliances help, although I still prefer the closer shave of a safety razor over an electric one. With grooming as with dressing, I seek "low maintenance." My haircut does not require styling gel or blow drying – just shampoo, rinse, towel dry, and a simple brushing into place. No change in deodorant application, and I've always used cologne sparingly.

Nail trimming is the most difficult with the loss of manual dexterity. I have both my fingernails and toenails trimmed professionally. Not a complete mani-pedi – just trimmed once every three weeks. My wife tried doing it for me, but after one attempt, we agreed that I should see a pro – less blood on the carpet and less stress on the marriage.

Toilet (acquired patterns – application layer)
Again, ladies, I can be of no help on this one and again, I'm sorry.

Gentlemen, since graduating from potty training, you have taken yourself in hand to *stand and deliver. Fagetaboudit.* Those days are gone. Have a seat. Otherwise, the day will come when, midstream, you'll suffer palsy tremors in your shootin' hand, and before you can let go, you'll have made extra work for yourself – mop the floor, shampoo the rug, paint the walls, retexture the ceiling, take a shower, do the laundry, and put on clean clothes. To make matters worse, manual dexterity (as noted earlier) when off your meds, is MIA. Manipulating timely extraction through at least two layers of access ports is often a struggle in itself. Save yourself the effort and embarrassment. Sit, *Ubu*, sit.

Having accepted that, there are still challenges. First, there's the task of drawer-dropping which involves a belt buckle or suspenders (please – not both), at least one button, a zipper, a shirttail, your trousers, and your underpants. If you're wearing a coat or jacket, remove it before you begin. If balance is a problem, brace yourself on something.

You may feel an urgent need to rush. **DON'T PANIC**. Relax. Stress and anxiety only make everything worse. Concentrate. **PICK UP YOUR FEET – SWING YOUR ARMS – CLOSE YOUR MOUTH – SWALLOW – BLINK – SMILE**. You've done this a million times. Simply reverse the steps from getting dressed. Your mind knows how your muscles are supposed to move. Concentrate. Steady, now – unbuckle, unbutton, unzip, drop 'em.

Next, you must negotiate the whole "standing-to-sitting" maneuver – difficult enough with conventional furniture; damn near impossible on the first try, targeting a portal. Remember the motto of the U.S. Navy *Seabees*: "*The difficult we do immediately. The impossible takes us a*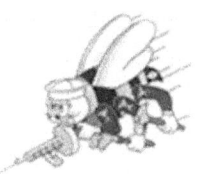

little while." Again, hang on to something. At home, you may as well swallow (without drooling or choking) your pride and get a walker. You'll need one, eventually. Public restroom handicapped stalls have hand rails. Very convenient.

When ready, you must deal with the task at hand. Incontinence has not (yet) been a problem, but the need is often sudden and urgent, creating panic. The bladder is a highly specialized muscle, and in the "off-med" rush and fumble to extract and/or sit, muscle control patterns may be inaccessible, resulting in premature emission. Frequent occurrence may indicate a need for disposable protection. It just *depends*. Be decisive.

Since you're already seated, it is appropriate to discuss solid waste emanations from the seventh planet. From hard constipation to loose diarrhea – you will experience the full range, with no discernable cause and effect. Regularity? Unless you're unusually lucky, it ain't happ'nin'. Again, the colon is just another highly specialized muscle. If the problem becomes severe, seek relief through your medical team.

What I want to share is the follow-up. While seated, the paper work may be difficult. If you can stand without making a mess and bend forward without falling (hang on to something), you may find that task less daunting. Flushable, pre-moistened wipes are a nice touch. I recommend them. Then there's the whole "pull up, tuck in, zip up, button up, buckle up" task. When you're off your meds, that can be a frustrating struggle, especially if extra tries are needed. Oh, yeah – *WASH YOUR HANDS.*

Intimacy (acquired patterns – application layer)
Ladies, again, I apologize for my gender-specific knowledge of this sensitive subject. I can only relate to *erectile dysfunction* as a man.

Guys, either PD, your meds, or both may cause your manly apparatus to "turtle in." Yes, chemistry can help, but use caution: check with your medical team. These blood-rushing, muscle-stiffening wonders can cause indigestion (for more than four hours), adversely interact with your PD meds, or put undue stress on your heart or kidneys. They may even cause your partner discomfort.

If you don't suffer any degraded performance from this malady, chalk it up in the *WIN* column and sally forth – or Betty third – or Marsha second – or whomever whenever. If, on the other hand, you're holding "*...a candle in the wind,*" you can try the blue diamond or one of its competing snake-oil compounds, under medical supervision, of course. If you and your partner experience no adverse side-effects, that is also a *WIN*. If you experience some discomfort, and you feel that the pleasure more than offsets the displeasure, take the *WIN* for "*...courage under fire.*" If nothing works – you can't tolerate the drugs, and you can't mount like a stallion, there are manipulations available that are beyond the scope of this discussion. In any case, don't mark it as a loss. Put it in the *WIN* bucket as "*one less miracle you have to perform.*" **IMPORTANT TIP**: CLOSE YOUR MOUTH and SWALLOW frequently. No matter how good you think you are or what moves you may have, nothing chills her mood quite like drooling on her face.

Sick days (acquired patterns – application layer)
You'll get the flu, a cold, or some other minor ailment that puts you on the 3-day DL. Stay down, Stay quiet. Drink liquids. Treat the illness the same as if you didn't have PD. Tell the Doc and the pharmacist what meds you take to avoid adverse drug interaction.

Smoking and illegal drugs (acquired patterns – application layer)
Seriously? Is this topic really necessary? Don't you have enough of a challenge without intentionally handicapping both your mind *and* your brain – to say nothing of what harm you are doing to your already disabled body? Really?

CHAPTER 8

Conclusion

James G. Parkinson, RCS, FGS (1755 – 1824)
The Docs' "First Contact" Communications
Orientation Classes
Finding a Cure
Persistence & Determination
Don't Panic

James G. Parkinson, *RCS, FGS* (1755 – 1824)

Champion of the Common Man – Compassionate Physician to the Suffering

Born, raised, and educated in London, where the celebrated apothecary, surgeon, explorer, paleontologist, and political activist – Dr. James Parkinson, of the *Royal College of Surgeons*, and a *Fellow of the Geological Society* – conducted his medical practices and organized his digging expeditions. A prolific author, he published numerous geological articles on the fossilized remains of several prehistoric creatures that he unearthed; plus his medical essays on Gout, Appendicitis, and of course – *The Shaking Palsy*.

Politically, Parkinson openly opposed the English nobility's dominion over the landless working class. He published many controversial essays touting the common causes of *universal suffrage* and the creation of a second parliamentary body consisting of elected Commoner representatives, to be known as the *House of Commons*. He secretly applauded the French rebels for dethroning their country's aristocracy, despite those acts which most Britons considered to be the worst kind of barbaric terrorism.

As the 18th century ended, the Brits were tired of war. A war with France ending with a treaty, followed by a war with France ending with a treaty, followed by a war with France ending with a treaty – on and **ON** – for *seven hundred years!* War with France landed on the American continent, lasting seven years and costing thousands of pounds to gain territory, only to see it forfeited in a more costly, five-year debacle in which His Majesty's invincible British Army lost the colonies to a traitorous band of common brigands.

From their standpoint, the French resented the English for favoring their mongrel Anglo-Saxon roots over their proud Norman heritage, driving on the wrong side of the road, and audaciously naming the straight separating the two countries, the *English* Channel.

Now, the French were killing each other, lopping off heads, including those of their Monarch and the Royal Family. For Parkinson to have publicly supported the French Revolution would have meant his risking social ostracism, professional banishment, and open confrontations with adversaries like Edmund Burke and Thomas Carlyle.

When Parkinson retired from his expeditionary globe-trotting, he settled in the North, concentrating on a different type of exploration – medical research. His *Essay on the Shaking Palsy* was an attempt to unify the field of medicine on a standard diagnosis and treatment. *Neurology* was just emerging as its own discipline, mapping the human brain.

It would be half-a-century before Dr. Jean-Martin Charcot, the "*Napoleon of neuro-science*," would give formal definition to the disease, supported by scientific research. One of his students, a young Austrian neurologist, Sigmund Freud, would ultimately map the human mind and propose that the brain and the mind are two distinct entities, not always compatible with one another. Parkinson christened the disorder, *Paralysis Agitans* (*Latin:* SHAKING PALSY). It was Charcot who renamed it – *Parkinson's disease*.

Such is the man's legacy – all of his geological and paleontological discoveries – all of his scientific and medical breakthroughs – along with his progressive social activism: fair treatment of Commoners, universal voting rights, and popular-based government reform – yet what **CAN** did *History* tie to this renowned humanitarian-physician-explorer-paleontologist-statesman's tail? For *Eternity* this debilitating, degenerative disease that callously eradicates the human mind by slowly ravaging the human brain will be tagged with his name – "*Maxime pravus cum ironiæ!*"

The Docs' "*First Contact*" Communications

Every field of endeavor has its own language – its own terminology. Anyone who knows anything about airplanes knows what "*VFR*" means. All serious baseball fans know what an "*RBI*" is. Neurology is no different. Neurology professionals speak their own lingo. That's fine for discussion among themselves, but when newly afflicted PD patients, unfamiliar with the jargon, are part of the discussion, they get very lost very quickly.

The first time a person hears the words *"Parkinson's disease"* applied to his brain is a terribly frightening, mind-numbing moment. Fear hijacks all capacity for rational thought. No amount of soft-spoken words or empathetic tone can allay that fear. The first questions in a new patient's mind are *"What's going to happen to me?"* *"How much time do I have?"* and *"Will I be in pain?"* Docs need to better prepare to respond to those fears.

Yes, everyone is different, but there are commonalities. Yes, the Docs are busy. They have a lot of patients. Their time is precious. Still, they need to allow extra time on the day that they first speak those frightening words to a newly afflicted patient. They also they need to listen. Rather than handing over a yellow sticky note with the *APDA* URL scrawled across it, they should hand out a comprehensive information packet.

Some people will want minute details. Others will be in denial. Neurology pros should be prepared with a range of responses in words that will help the patient comprehend his situation and get passed the emotion, so he can begin to deal with Parkinson's rationally. Schedule an early visit with the care giver. Some patients may need counseling. In addition to prescribing therapy, refer them to support groups with others who have faced the terrors, have overcome them, and are capable to mentor the newbies.

Orientation Classes

After having six stents inserted into my coronary arteries, the cardiologist enrolled me in Physical Therapy group sessions which, along with exercise, provided educational group lectures on heart disease, risk factors, and changing our lifestyles to strengthen and protect our hearts following surgery. Such orientation training for new newly afflicted Parkinson's patients would be most appropriate. Topics that should be included –

1. Parkinson's terminology;
2. brain composition – specifically, those brain components associated with PD;

3. brain chemistry – specifically, those brain chemicals associated with PD;
4. the *Unified Parkinson's Disease Rating Scale* (*UPDRS*) – how it's scored, typical intervals, and what the cumulative total score indicates;
5. the benefits of a neurological/psychological examination;
6. long-term prognosis – timing, stage progression (e.g. dementia, declining abilities);
7. fatal complications – DVT, PE, pulmonary aspiration, and fatal falls;
8. the importance of a positive attitude – mind vs. brain & combating fear with facts;
9. personality and temperament – potential changes as the disease progresses;
10. care givers – how their role will change as the disease progresses;
11. support network team – members, roles, and responsibilities;
12. symptoms – form, severity, response tactics, treatment, et al;
13. coping tactics – planning, developing, implementing, adjusting, adapting, improvising;
14. diet & nutrition – antioxidants, proteins, caffeine, alcohol in moderation, & ***ice cream***;
15. medication – what it is, what it does, typical dosages, timing, gradual resistance;
16. therapy – speech, occupational, physical, psychological counseling;
17. exercise – supervised or self-managed, it should be professionally prescribed;
18. mental acuity – read, write, *THINK*, imagine, do head math;
19. sleep – get it, you'll need it;
20. driving – Dude (Dudette), three words…
21. self-Heimlich – how to save your own life: learn it, practice it (supervised); and
22. protective falling – how to save your own life: learn it, practice it (supervised).

Finding a Cure

When a catastrophic system failure occurs in the IT world, the first priority is to fully restore stable system operation. Restoration often involves "*Band-Aid®* fixes" that only remedy individual symptoms, to enable a return to service, while a full understanding of what caused the failure remains unknown. Once the operation is stabilized, a comprehensive, system-wide examination known as *Root Cause Analysis* (*RCA*) is undertaken to determine what underlying factor(s) led to the failure. From this analysis, the root cause *remedial action* can be planned, designed, developed, and implemented with the intent of avoiding repeat failures. Don't simply treat the symptom. Resolve the underlying problem. You know – *"Give a man a fish..." "Teach a man to fish..."* et cetera.

Parkinson's disease results from a lack of the brain chemical, *dopamine*, which is produced by specific brain cells called *dopaminergic neurons* located in the *substantia nigra* (don't ask – just take a deep breath and go with it). *Why do the dopaminergic neurons stop producing dopamine?* **Because they die.** *What kills them? That,* for the moment, is the show stopper. Even if we should find the dopaminergic neuron *Cause of Death*, there is no guarantee of that being the root cause of Parkinson's. That is simply the next step. There may be more (many more?) steps hiding behind that one. Without live dopaminergic neuron cells to analyze, we have no test tissue on which to conduct three crucial analyses: *Cause of Death*, *Remedial Action*, and *Preventive Measures*. Sources for obtaining test cells are limited.

Theoretically, actual cells could be harvested from a living human brain, but that would be lethal for both the cells and the donor brain, so Hippocrates squelched that idea. Another source is to regenerate dopaminergic neurons from *stem cells*. The generic foundation for all human tissue, stem cells contain the body's basic cell structure and the potential for transforming into almost any of the innumerable types of human specialized cells. Known sources of *autologous* (from one's own body) adult stem cells in humans are bone marrow, lipid cells, and blood. However, dopaminergic neurons develop very early in human gestation cycle, and these stem cells develop beyond where they can regress into dopamine-producing cells.

Stem cells can be harvested from an individual's umbilical cord blood at birth and preserved for use by that individual, later in life. However, the cost of such a procedure is well beyond what most people can afford, and since its effectiveness in PD analysis is unproven, it is unlikely that healthcare insurers will cover such a costly experimental procedure. Besides, for sufferers my age, that procedure is not an option. Our parents didn't have the foresight to harvest and store any of our umbilical blood stem cells.

Hey! It was 1947. *Who knew?*

In the final analysis, the stem cells that hold the most promise of evolving into dopaminergic neurons are those harvested from a newly conceived human embryo. Since harvesting human embryonic stem cells destroys the donor embryo, an irreconcilable moral impasse blocks the procedure. (OK, *Pro-Lifers & Pro-Choicers* – turn it up & bring it.) Even if the ovum and sperm are donated separately and artificially inseminated under laboratory conditions outside a human womb, for the expressed purpose of harvesting embryonic stem cells, the moral dilemma remains: *"Are we creating human life, only to terminate that life, all in the name of medical research?"* No joy. The answer to that question is well above my pay grade. As I said – it's a show stopper.

Persistence & Determination

> *"Nothing in this world can take the place of persistence. Talent will not; nothing is more common than unsuccessful men with talent. Genius will not; unrewarded genius is almost a proverb. Education will not; the world is full of educated derelicts. Persistence and Determination alone are omnipotent. The slogan 'Press On!' has solved and always will solve the problems of the human race."*
> — CALVIN COOLIDGE

I've just spent however many hours that you've spent reading this book coaching you on waging war with Parkinson's disease and its symptoms. Time for true confessions: it is far easier to commit this stuff to paper than it is to apply it persistently, day in and day out. There will be days when getting out of bed will be a daunting task. If you went to bed, or did you flop into the recliner for the third straight night while wearing the same clothes for three days and nights? There will be days when cognitive effort will consist of deciding which TV show to watch. There will be days (weeks) when your home's exercise room is no more than the room where the exercise equipment is stored.

Contending with Parkinson's is **HARD WORK**. Daily mind-over-brain victories require vigilance, dedication, commitment, consistency, and determination – *Persistent Determination* – **PD**. You'll get tired. You'll get bitchy. You'll stubbornly dig in your heels. You'll want to give in. Been there – done that. Trust me: every time you get lazy and fail to put forth the effort –*YOUR BRAIN WINS*.

Don't Panic

> "*If you are going through Hell, keep going.*"
> — WINSTON CHURCHILL

> "*We have nothing to fear but fear itself.*"
> — FRANKLIN D. ROOSEVELT

There you have it. You have Parkinson's. I have Parkinson's. Seven million people have Parkinson's. It won't kill you. Some complication of the disease may kill you, but who knows? Everybody dies. Nobody knows how or when they're going to die – *FAGETABOUDIT*. You can add years to your life and minimize the adverse impact of PD to yourself and your loved ones by facing fear and overcoming it rationally. Fear is the shrouded enemy. Unveil it in the light of reason. You're in a life-long war for time: your [*PD*] *P*arkinson's *D*iseased *BRAIN* vs. your [*PD*] *P*ersistently *D*etermined *MIND*. Listen to me – I know. By now, you know I know. Establish a routine and **WORK IT** – faithfully.

1. PICK UP YOUR FEET - SWING YOUR ARMS - CLOSE YOUR MOUTH - SWALLOW - BLINK - SMILE;
2. be nice;
3. take your meds – on time – as prescribed;
4. establish your support network; but
5. do as much as you can to take care of yourself;
6. practice your tactics, especially protective falling and self-Heimlich Maneuver;

7. exercise your body and your mind;
8. *THINK*: about stuff – before you speak – before you act – before you move;
9. engage with life – stay active – stay productive;
10. <u>DO NOT</u> drive in an unmedicated state – FYI, Colorado is NOT a medicated State;
11. laugh – have fun;
12. read – write – sing – dance – work – play – GO FISHING;
13. get a good night's sleep;
14. count your blessings;
15. do good works – help others less fortunate than yourself;
16. cherish the time you spend with those who care for and about you; and
17. beware of the **DARK SIDE** – fear, paranoia, and self-pity.

Remember, the strategies and tactics in this book work on my symptoms. They may or may not work on yours. You must tailor your tactics to fit your circumstances. Analyze your symptoms for impact, severity, duration, frequency, initiators, and response to medication. Share that information with your Docs. Use the tactics in this book as a starting point, then *IMPROVISE* and *ADAPT* to *OVERCOME* each of your symptoms.

Never give up. Never quit. Keep the faith. Now that you've read this book, read it again – and again. Don't put it on the shelf. Keep it handy. There's stuff you didn't get the first time – stuff you glossed over as your eyes glazed over. Go back and dig into it. Keep your mind busy and challenged with the hard stuff in this book. **PICK UP YOUR FEET – SWING YOUR ARMS – CLOSE YOUR MOUTH – SWALLOW – BLINK – SMILE – BE NICE.** Most importantly – **DON'T PANIC.**

Throughout these pages, I have shared uplifting quotations to help boost your spirits. You're in for a rough patch. You'll fight the good fight every minute of every day. Your mind can only wage its perpetual battle with your brain by using tactics of another PD – *Persistent Determination*, but eventually, your damaged brain will prevail and assert its malevolent control of your body. I saved my favorite quotation for last. If you're not a fan of legendary four-legged athletes with names like *Gallant Fox*, *Omaha*, *Whirlaway*, and *Citation*, who were ridden by legendary two-legged athletes with names like *Longden*, *Shoemaker*, and *Arcaro*; you won't recognize the author – but take his words to heart.

> "*When the One Great Scorer comes to mark against your name,*
> *He'll mark not that you won or lost – but how you played the game.*"
> – GRANTLAND RICE
> *THE TUMULT AND THE SHOUTING*

God speed.

Acknowledgements

- The medical and administrative staff in the U.S. Department of Veterans Affairs, Nebraska/Western Iowa Healthcare System – Omaha's Veterans' Hospital for providing compassionate, quality healthcare to Nebraska and Iowa U.S. Military veterans.
- Dr. John Bertoni, M.D., Ph.D., Director – Parkinson's Disease Program and Professor of Neurological Sciences, University of Nebraska Medical Center for his dedicated leadership in the management of my case as the Attending Neurologist at the Omaha VA Hospital. Dr. Bertoni is a nationally recognized authority on Parkinson's disease with more than 40 years' experience. The author of over a dozen publications on PD and its impact, he graciously offered to write the *Forward* for this book. He has been a continual inspiration, an empathetic guide, and a relentless source of encouragement.
- Dr. Dennis Molfese, Ph.D. – Mildred Francis Thompson Professor of Psychology at the University of Nebraska-Lincoln and Founding Director Emeritus of UN-L's Center for Brain Biology and Behavior which investigates questions related to the brain's involvement in cognitive processes (e.g. *learning* and *language*) across the lifespan. Dr. Molfese helped me to understand, from my lay person's perspective, how the brain's different motor and cognitive functions are adversely affected by Parkinson's disease.
- Dr. Julie Honaker, Ph.D. – Associate Professor, Department of Special Education and Communication Disorders, University of Nebraska-Lincoln. She teaches graduate courses on vestibular and balance

disorder assessment and management. Her Ph.D. in Audiology is from the University of Cincinnati. She most recently completed a Post-Doctorate Fellowship at the Mayo Clinic. Dr. Honaker has a passion for the clinical assessment and rehabilitation of balance disorder patients. She kept me from stumbling when I was writing the sections on PD *Balance* and *Mobility*.

- Dr. Rebecca Reilly, M.D. – Geriatrician with Methodist Health Systems in Omaha, Nebraska. Some medical practitioners are Doctors and others are *Physicians*. You have to know Becky Reilly to know the difference. Some people age gracefully, others grow old kicking and screaming. Dr. Reilly's compassionate care gently guides her patients toward graceful aging and fulfilled lifestyles. Her insight relating to the unique medical challenges faced by the elderly was invaluable.

- Anne Potter, PT at the Sue Jeffrey Physical Therapy Clinic in Lincoln, Nebraska – my *Protective Falling* and *Self-Administered Heimlich* collaborator. She supervised and recorded results as I – helmeted and padded – tried various protective techniques during a number of test falls. She ran the tests. I was the crash-test dummy. We also spent quality time while I attempted to eject ping-pong balls from my mouth by thrusting my fist up and into my abdomen. Thank you, Henry Heimlich.

- David Russell – my editorial advisor who knows when I need leadership and when I need to wander; my former boss who knew when to manage and when to simply clear the path; and my long-time friend who has always had time to listen. Dave helped me stay on topic and steer my rants and rambles into meaningful, dialogue. An accomplished author in his own right, Dave has patiently guided me in crafting my wild-hare, thinking and my left-field logic into something that people may actually want to read.

- Deborah Spidle – my IT guru, my trusted colleague, my valued friend. She is my subject matter expert, patient tutor, and tireless fact checker on all things technical. Her forté is delivering elegant automated solutions to meet complex requirements for integrated banking and transaction processing systems on time and within budget. A master of her craft and a lady in the truest sense of the word, she is unflappable, unimpeachable, and unequalled in a profession that is awash with testosterone.

- Frank Bracken – Douglas County Veterans' Service Officer, American Legion (Nebraska). Frank is one of those dedicated, indispensable, procedural-unsung-hero, back-office experts that the world simply cannot do without. A Viet Nam veteran, himself, his compassion, commitment, and effectiveness at cutting through all of the VA's bureaucratic red tape is unparalleled. Without Frank, the veterans of Douglas County, Nebraska would be in a serious Hurt Locker. Respectfully, we SALUTE him.

- My children, Melissa Baumbick, Laura Jennings, and Cody Currey – who, despite my inconsistent parenting, have grown to be wonderful people of fine character. Credit your mothers. Thank you for standing by me, even when I wasn't there to stand by.

- Kemper Wilkins – my brudder from anudder mudder. The man I look up to (literally – he's 6'1" and I'm 5'9") and wish that I could be more like. A two-tour Viet Nam veteran who has had his own demons to vanquish, he is the kind of man whose dignity and exceptional character are abundantly evident in five fine individuals – his children, and *their* children. Without his example to follow, this book would not have been written.

- Sheilah Widhalm – my beautiful sister. Her brother was an only child, until she "found" me. That is another story for another time – definitely Oprah Winfrey stuff. Thank you for lighting the darkness with your kindness and your patient understanding.

- John Moragues, MSW, Major, USAF [Ret] – the only one of my boyhood friends from 58th Street who has stayed in contact. Another brother in arms during the Viet Nam War, John made a career of the Air Force. He went on to become a dedicated social worker and, ultimately, Associate Professor of Social Work and Distance Education Coordinator at Newman University in Colorado Springs. Having known me for nearly all my life, John helps me stay grounded in reality whenever my Roddenberry-esque IQ wants to go "…*where no man has gone before!*" John is always at the ready with the answers to the hard questions like, "*Is God a Democrat or a Republican?*"

- Lori Richter. Tami Whitney, and Levi Schreck – three close friends whose opinions I value. Younger than I, they have that rare quality that equates wisdom with age and experience. All three excellent communicators, they helped me to convey clear, concise, grammatically correct and properly punctuated concepts.
- Saving the very best for last – my wife, Kim, who gets her own chapter in the book.

Resources

American Parkinson's Disease
Association
135 Parkinson Avenue
Staten Island, NY 10305
Phone: 800-223-2732 or
718-981-8001
Fax: 718-981-4399
www.apdaparkinson.org

National Parkinson's Foundation
200 SE 1st Street, Suite 800
Miami, Florida 33131
Toll-free Helpline: 1-800-473-4636)
Fax: (305) 537-9901
www.parkinson.org

The Michael J. Fox Foundation for
Parkinson's Research
Grand Central Station
P.O. Box 4777
New York, NY 10163-4777
1-800-708-7644
www.michaeljfox.org

U.S. Department of Veterans'
Affairs
810 Vermont Avenue, NW
Washington, DC 20420
1-800-827-1000
www.va.gov

American Legion
700 N. Pennsylvania St.
P.O. Box 1055
Indianapolis, IN 46206
Telephone: (317) 630-1200
Fax: (317) 630-1223
www.legion.org

Viet Nam Veterans of America
8719 Colesville Rd., Suite 100
Silver Spring, Maryland 20910
1-800-882-1316
301-585-4000
301-585-0519 – fax
www.vva.org

YMCA of the USA
101 N Wacker Drive
Chicago, IL 60606
1-800-872-9622
www.ymca.net

LSVT Global, Inc.
3323 N. Campbell Ave, Suite 5
Tucson, AZ 85719
Toll Free: 1-888-438-5788
Phone: 1-520-867-8838
Fax: 1-520-867-8839
www.lsvtglobal.com

www.ingramcontent.com/pod-product-compliance
Lightning Source LLC
Chambersburg PA
CBHW071210280526
45787CB00002B/636